YOKE

My Yoga of Self-Acceptance

JESSAMYN STANLEY

Workman Publishing
New York

Sutras excerpted from *The Yoga Sutras of Patanjali:*
Translations and commentary by Sri Swami Satchidananda © 2012
by Satchidananda Ashram—Yogaville, Inc.
(Integral Yoga Publications, Buckingham, Virginia)

Library of Congress Cataloging-in-Publication Data
Names: Stanley, Jessamyn, author.
Title: Yoke : my yoga of self-acceptance / Jessamyn Stanley ;
cover illustration by Shanée Benjamin ; interior illustrations by Joelle Avelino.
Description: First. | New York : Workman Publishing, [2021] |
Identifiers: LCCN 2021003537 | ISBN 9781523505210 (paperback) |
ISBN 9781523505210 (ebook)
Subjects: LCSH: Hatha yoga. | Exercise. | Mind and body therapies.
Classification: LCC RA781.7 .S724 2021 | DDC 613.7/046—dc23
LC record available at https://lccn.loc.gov/2021003537

ISBN 978-1-5235-0521-0

Design by Becky Terhune
Cover illustration by Shanée Benjamin
Interior illustrations by Joelle Avelino

Workman books are available at special discounts when purchased in bulk for
premiums and sales promotions as well as for fundraising or educational use.
Special editions or book excerpts can also be created to specification.
For details, contact the Special Sales Director at
specialmarkets@workman.com.

Workman Publishing Co., Inc.
225 Varick Street
New York, NY 10014-4381
workman.com

WORKMAN is a registered trademark of
Workman Publishing Co., Inc.

Printed in the United States of America
First printing June 2021

10 9 8 7 6 5 4 3 2 1

For everyone who
walked so I can run,
but especially
Tangela Michelle.

CONTENTS

FOREWORD

I wrote most of the essays in this book before 2020, before COVID-19, when Breonna Taylor and George Floyd were still with us.

Every day, more of what we know falls apart. The dream of America is burning.

Everyone is scared of what'll happen next. No one is immune to the fear. And everyone's fear is valid.

Pull up a chair, your fear is welcome here. You are welcome here, exactly as you are. You don't need to change anything or do anything differently. You don't need to hide anything or pretend that something's not there. All your sadness, all your anger, all your doubt, all your frustration, all your confusion. It's all welcome here. All of you is welcome here.

The part where it's uncomfortable. The part where you're ashamed of yourself. The part where you say the wrong thing and piss someone off. The part where you're stuck in the same place and don't know what to do next.

The universe is forcing us to quit with the bullshit and to show each other how we really feel. But when you forgive the smelliness and accept the ugliness of it all, what lies beneath is just as beautiful as anything else. Just as beautiful as a decaying flower, a rose on the last day of its life.

Have hope in yourself, in your family, and in your children. We have seen worse than this. We will see worse than this. There is always hope, even when there may be worse to come.

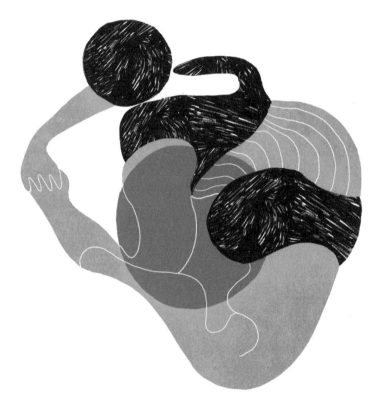

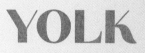

1.2 - "The restraint of the modifications of the mind-stuff is Yoga." (Satchidananda, 3)[1]

1.14 - "Practice becomes firmly grounded when well attended to for a long time, without break and in all earnestness." (Satchidananda, 19)

1.13 - "It means you become eternally watchful, scrutinizing every thought, every word, and every action." (Satchidananda, 18)

---

1 Sutras excerpted from Sri Swami Satchidananda, translation with commentary added.

Okay, so it's after midnight a few months after the release of *Every Body Yoga*, my first book. I'm wide awake in my home office and knee-deep in a Wikipedia wormhole when a Gmail notification BLOOPs into view.

For the record, I hate push notifications. They're such a buzzkill. Sometimes they're helpful, but then again, so are mansplainers. And just like a mansplainer, a push notification is much more likely to irreparably fuck with your day.

Anyway, this particular notification was from someone who'd read *Every Body Yoga* and was *so deeply affected by it* that she felt compelled to send me an email. In the middle of the night. A complete stranger sent me an email in the middle of the night.

Sigh.

In my experience, unsolicited late-night correspondence from a complete stranger is rarely a good thing. I've found that the fine print on being a fat, Black, queer yoga teacher in a predominantly thin, White, and *very* straight yoga industry is that there are just as many people who are inspired by you as there are with a strong desire for you to shut the fuck up. I pressed my palms together and prayed for the best.

Apparently, the messenger was a freelance copy editor soliciting her services on my next literary project because, as a yoga practitioner herself, she was appalled by a very specific typo in *Every Body Yoga*.

Uh-oh.

I snatched up my nearest copy of *Every Body Yoga* and 'bout got a paper cut in pursuit of the page she'd referenced. My heart stopped. Right there, on page twenty-fucking-nine, I'd accidentally defined the Sanskrit word *yoga* as meaning "to *yolk*."

Girl, I 'bout fell out.

I'd MEANT to use the word *yoke*, meaning "to join together." Yoga means *to yoke*, as in, to join together the light and dark of life, the good and the bad. Yoke, as in, "let's yoke these cattle together." To yoke is to marry breath, thought, and movement, to connect the body, mind, and spirit. To yoke is to explore the meaning of balance.

This definition stands in stark contrast to the definition of *yolk*, which means "the yellow food storage sphere composing a substantial percentage of an egg's interior." This was a glaring typo, certainly worthy of criticism. I couldn't believe that after dozens of drafts and round after round of edits, I'd failed to notice such an obvious mistake.

Now, I've gotta be honest with you, especially if you and I are gonna have a real relationship and not just be on some bullshit. Straight up, my knee-jerk reaction to that email was to pop shots. How dare this bitch try to call me out? And in a passive-aggressive, after-midnight, stranger-danger-ass email, no less! If she *was* in fact a copy editor (and not merely a bored, lonely internet troll nursing a vendetta, as I secretly suspected), then she must understand that typos are to be expected in a work of any substantial size. Before long, I was shit-talking and verbally drop-kicking this bitch all the way into next week.

But once my Mars in Cancer cleared the scene, my anger flushed to red-hot embarrassment. I was seized by a need to wake up my editor so we could run risk assessment options on possibly reprinting *Every Body Yoga*'s entire run.

Instead, I did something that's gradually become my Pavlovian response to stress and anxiety. I sighed, closed my eyes, walked over to my yoga mat, and unrolled it right in the middle of my office.

I didn't start practicing handstands or any acrobatic shit like that. I just sat down and closed my eyes.

I didn't tell myself, "Time to meditate!"

I didn't start a timer or practice a specific breath-work technique.

I just sat down and focused my attention on trying to breathe. Steady, in and out through the nose.

I didn't try to *stop* thinking about what was stressing me out. I actually did the exact opposite. I let my Virgo rising run wild and allowed myself to consider every nook and cranny of my anxiety. Instead of trying to kick out my inner critic, I made space at the table. And the whole time, as my mind raked my angst over the coals, I just tried to breathe.

At first, my breath came shallow and timid, tinted with uncertainty. But as my body submitted to its whim, my breath stood up straighter and rolled back its shoulders. It started to take itself seriously and believe in itself. My breath whistled around the branches of my anxiety and I found myself softening like forgotten butter. And, gradually, I began to see the surface of what had *actually* pissed me off.

It wasn't the typo.

It wasn't the email or its sender.

It was my imposter syndrome. The imposter syndrome I'd felt ever since I'd posted my first yoga picture on Instagram. The feeling that I didn't know enough about yoga to participate in a mainstream conversation about it. The feeling that I could never read enough books, that I could never take enough classes, that I could never work on postures hard enough. I'd managed to publish a whole-ass book about yoga before my thirtieth birthday and I subconsciously believed that every yoga practitioner and teacher knew how unqualified I was for the task. I doubted my ability and assumed that everyone else did as well.

As a social media influencer-cum-yoga teacher, I regularly feign confidence. Much as I try as to fight it, projecting confidence is part of the influencer job description. Yet all it took was one loose-lipped email from a complete stranger about a singular typo to crush my projection of confidence.

Cornered by shame and inadequacy, I saw how I spent most of my days and much of my energy desperately trying to *outrun* that truth. On my yoga mat, forlorn in my crab shell and weary of the chase, I stopped running. Instead of continuing to run, I embraced my fear of myself, and I began unbandaging wounds that I've carried as long as I can remember.

All wounds need to breathe, no matter how painful or smelly. Even the wounds you'd rather keep hidden.

Yoga links the deepest and most conflicted aspects of myself. The light and the dark. The bad and the good. The ups and the downs. It's both a process and a destination, both a question and an answer.

I turned twenty-five in the summer of 2012 and dropped out of my arts management MFA program a month before my birthday, a decision that mostly scared the shit outta me. I needed a change, and a new town seemed like as good a place as any to find one, so I loaded up my car and moved from Winston-Salem to Durham, North Carolina. My new girlfriend, S, had just moved to Durham, and even though we both felt it was too early in our relationship for cohabitation, neither of us could afford to live on our own. Plus, we were each other's only friend in Durham, so we agreed it'd be better to stick with the devil you know.

For the first bit, S and I shared a tiny twin bed in an even tinier apartment owned by two middle-aged codependent Black dykes that we code-named Big Bear and little bear. While Big B and lil b spooned on the queen next door, S and I slept like a seal pod on a bed built for a teenager. Two adult fatties in a twin bed, even a twin XL, ain't nobody's idea of a long-term solution. And certainly not in a poorly air-conditioned prefab apartment in North Carolina's armpit at the height of summer.

S and I brought to our relationship nearly twenty combined years of lesbian codependency. None of it, not one stinking year, had adequately prepped us for the ugly reality of sharing that teeny-weeny bed. Not even my most "lezbehonest" boarding school memories were proper training. After a while, we'd just alternate between one of us sleeping on the floor while the other one spread out like a starfish on the bed. As for storage space, my car was my closet, leaving me one carjacking away from the loss of all my worldly possesions.

But by the time S and I got settled in an apartment that fit both our bodies and our wallets, we had bigger shit on our minds than limited closet space. Within the first year or so of living together, S's brother Richard, my aunt Tiriah, and my grandma Marvella all died.

First up was Aunt Tiriah, the aunt who taught me how to bathe myself and who caught me getting fresh with the boy next door. Aunt Tiriah always understood me, especially when my mom didn't.

Maybe you don't believe in dying of a broken heart, but I think my Grandma's grief over Aunt Tiriah's sudden passing brought on her own. The diabetes she'd successfully managed for at least a decade somehow became unmanageable after Aunt Tiriah died.

And just a few months after his twenty-first birthday, Richard was murdered in a hit-and-run car accident. S and I had literally just seen him—I swear he'd been by the house not even a few weeks before we got the call. His was the kind of death that makes people tut-tut because what else is there to say when an intelligent, beautiful, witty, creative, and incredibly kind person who just turned twenty-one dies senselessly and far too soon?

Their deaths left a void that S and I were unsure how to fill. I thought God might be the answer, but I had my doubts. I was raised in a devout Bahá'í household, but I'd drifted from the religiosity of my childhood. Retreating to its complicated embrace in the wake of death felt disingenuous to me. I was drifting and felt unsure of where, or even how, to pivot.

I'd maintained a regular Bikram yoga practice for about a year before moving to Durham, and it had drastically helped my mental health as things fell apart in my grad program. My budget had been way too tight for the drop-in rates at my local studio, but I was able to participate in a work-study program that allowed me to help out with studio housekeeping in exchange for free yoga classes.

As soon as I got settled in Durham, I sought out similar work-study opportunities at every yoga studio I could find. I was disappointed to find that Durham's yoga scene was much more crowded and competitive than Winston-Salem's. Most of the studios I solicited didn't have work-study programs at all. Those that did had over-flowing waitlists. I added my name but held little hope.

For several weeks, I didn't practice yoga at all and I didn't miss it one bit. I figured it was just another hobby I could let fall to the wayside. Like the summer I dabbled in oil painting or the years I spent collecting vintage fondue pots and early editions of *The Joy of Cooking*. I didn't really give a fuck about the mind, body, spirit connection. I'd yet to make the connection between yoga and my improved mental health, so I didn't really value its presence in my life. I thought dissatisfaction was a hallmark of life and, if anything, yoga had been a distraction from reality.

Then one day, out of the blue, I unrolled my yoga mat on the singular strip of empty hardwood floor in our cramped living room. The mat was handed down to me by my Daddy. A longtime Pilates nut, he gave me his old mat when I started going to yoga classes. His muscles were molded into the PVC, which stunk of both our sweat. It may not have been much more than a dust ruffle between me and the floorboards, but at least it was a *little* cushion for the pushin'.

At first I just sat there on my mat, unsure of how to go forward without a teacher. I was accustomed to following the guidance of yoga generalissimos. Without a teacher to follow, I was paralyzed by performance anxiety.

I wondered, "Am I even *allowed* to practice yoga without supervision?"

"Of course," said the Voice.

I didn't know where the Voice was coming from, but it sounded very steady and solid, like a deeply assured version of myself. And it sounded way too confident to contradict.

I stood up and walked to the top of my mat. I rolled back my shoulders, interlaced my fingers beneath my chin, and started practicing Bikram yoga's iconic breath-work invocation. It felt a little weird to practice without any supervision. A bit freeing, a bit scary. Like crossing the street without holding my mom's hand or riding my bike without training wheels. But once I got going, I still found myself awaiting further instructions.

As if on cue, the Voice began reciting every posture I'd mentally stored from the Bikram sequence. The Voice couldn't remember every single alignment cue that my Bikram teachers had ever uttered, but it remembered enough.

With gentle but firm benevolence, the Voice reminded me to keep my fingers interwoven with my thumbs rested against the thin skin that protects my throat. It reminded me to soften the very back of my gullet, inhaling and exhaling deeper with each successive breath. The Voice reminded me to treat each breath like my last.

I was *so* relieved to hear the Voice.

I held hands with the Voice and allowed the Voice to guide my body into action.

The Voice reminded me of every yoga pose I enjoyed in the Bikram sequence, even the ones I hated. In the privacy of our tiny apartment, furnished with our cat's hair and our complications, I rolled and curled and bent myself into shapes I'd been too timid to attempt when surrounded by other practitioners. And in those postures, I found myself trying harder and going further than I ever had before.

I began to notice the difference between who I am in the privacy of my own identity and who I choose to be in front of other people. I'm always afraid of offending other people or being too much, too big, taking up too much space, making too many sounds, being too hard to handle or too much to control. I began to see how much I restrain myself in public, making myself small and trying not to be noticed. But at home, I found myself contorting and emitting sounds I'd never had the confidence to express in public. I stopped apologizing for being loud and granted myself permission to take up space.

At home, everything was on the table. I could wear my underwear, smoke weed, and share meditative breaths with my cat. It didn't matter that I only knew a few postures. Instead of going my usual route of obsessing over everything I *didn't* know, I focused all my energy on the eight to ten poses that I *did* know. Instead of trying to know it all, I just let myself know what I know.

It's been nearly ten years, and I've gone from practicing in my living room to practicing in ad campaigns for brands like adidas and Amazon. The transition from yoga practitioner to yoga professional has left me feeling very conflicted. It's made me critique and analyze why I even started practicing yoga in the first place. When I started practicing yoga, my physical body reigned supreme over my subtle, or spiritual, body. My yoga may have started out being about practicing poses, but dealing with my mental and emotional baggage is the *real* yoga.

Classical yogic texts like *Hatha Yoga Pradipika* barely discuss postural practice at all because poses are really just one component of a yoga practice. The poses that have become symbolic of American yoga are really an amalgamation of Classical yogic postures combined with European calisthenics, Indian weightlifting, and other forms of kinesthetic movement, much of it developed and popularized in the nineteenth and twentieth centuries.

There are a lot of important differences between Classical yoga and American yoga. Classical yoga can be found at the root of Hinduism, Buddhism, Jainism, and a number of other spiritual and cultural practices. It's been practiced for thousands of years, whereas American yoga has only been active since the turn of the twentieth century, when teachers like Swami Vivekananda traveled to the United States from India to spread the practice of yoga. In the century since, American yoga lineages have proliferated across the globe.

At this point, American yoga studios, classes, and teachers can be found in just about every earthly crevice.

I wouldn't be surprised at all to find out that somebody's teaching yoga on research vessels in the Antarctic Circle. If I close my eyes, I can almost see it: a gaggle of scientists bedecked in monogrammed Patagonia, flowing through downward facing dog on snowy ship decks while colonies of bemused sea lions and penguins look on from their ice rafts, trying to figure out precisely why Homo sapiens are always doing the absolute Most.

There are almost as many styles of American yoga as there are practitioners on this planet, and most of them emphasize postural practice over spiritual practice. Like me, most American yoga practitioners pray at the church of Lululemon rather than engage with deeper yogic inquiry of the subtle body. And then, when American yoga practitioners *do* try to engage on a deeper level, we end up appropriating South Asian iconography and symbology and just generally embarrassing ourselves.

You don't have to appropriate South Asian culture to deepen your yoga practice. All you have to do is apply the lessons and techniques that you learn on your yoga mat to the daily project of living. I call it the *yoga of everyday life*.

In chair pose, you don't just sink your hips low and hope for the best. You have to engage every part of your body to make that shit happen. You have to root into your feet, dig into your core, engage your thighs, and wake up your toes. You have to try to fall down backward while still remaining upright. You have to learn to bend so you don't break.

The yoga of everyday life is the same thing. It's finding within life's shittiest moments the same flexibility, strength, grounding energy, and core awareness that you find in extended hand to big toe pose or headstand. This is yoga without accessories, a yoga you can practice without ever stepping on a mat.

When someone cuts you off in traffic and you resist the urge to road rage on them? That's yoga. Even if you *do* road rage on them, that's still yoga.

When your estranged parent rolls back into your life out of the blue after being gone for years and you're forced to deal with decades of trauma, that's yoga.

When someone you love dies and you find a way to (somehow) keep your head above water, that's yoga.

When you give birth to a whole-ass human being and then parent them for the rest of their life, that's yoga.

That time your kid called you a bitch in the middle of a crowded shopping center and you resisted the urge to abandon them on the spot? That was yoga.

When you accept your faults and the faults of others, that's yoga.

Yoga is to yoke. You yoke when you find a reason to get out of bed in the morning. You yoke when you peel yourself off the pavement after your heart's been broken (again). You yoke when you manage to keep moving in spite of being completely overwhelmed. You're always yoking, all the time.

My yoking ain't about anybody but me, and I can't

continue to wither under imposter syndrome until other people cosign my self-worth. I can only ever try to know myself and be present to my own divinity. I'm the only one who will ever know me, and I'm enough. Imposter syndrome is a distraction from the work at hand.

My yoga has many intersections and edges because, like the universe, I'm always unfolding. My yoga is finding out what it means to be a Black queer woman in a world that doesn't want me to be. It's holding space for when I've been assaulted, even when I'd rather hide my pain at the bottom of a bottle or a box. It's questioning my pursuit of power. It's coming to terms with a God of my *own* understanding, not a God that's been chosen for me. My yoga will probably eventually offend you. I mean, it offends *me*.

But yoga isn't about feeling only the happy emotions. It's about feeling *all* the emotions. Even when the emotion du jour is anger. One of the hardest things for me to accept is that not everyone will agree with or like how I've chosen to accept myself. I'm still that girl who wants the popular kids to like her. And when the popular kids don't understand where I'm coming from or they get angry at me for refusing to swim in the mainstream, I have to accept that, too. I have to accept being disliked and misunderstood because being disliked and misunderstood has more to do with how the popular kids feel about themselves than how I feel about me.

I can be disliked and be myself at the same time.

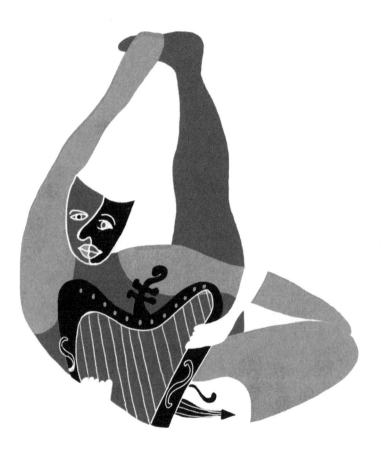

I'M NOT ME

1.3 - "Then the Seer (Self) abides in Its own nature." (Satchidananda, 6)

1.4 - "At other times [the Self appears to] assume the forms of the mental modifications." (Satchidananda, 7)

"But without any identifications, who are you? Have you ever thought about it? When you really understand that, you will see we are all the same. If you detach yourself completely from all the things you have identified yourself with, you realize yourself as the pure 'I.' In that pure 'I' there is no difference between you and me." (Satchidananda, 8)

"Remember that the body is not the experience. Life is experienced by the mind through the body. The body is only a vehicle." (Satchidananda, 92)

"A yogi should always keep this in mind. Teaching yoga is not like teaching history or geometry. Teachers must impart a life force—a little current—into others. How can they do this if they are weak, if they have rundown, discharged batteries? So keep your batteries full of energy." (Satchidananda, 130)

Practicing yoga feels like digging an instrument out of myself. It's all very *Walking Dead*. It's like I'm pulling an instrument from my organs, something I've never seen before and have no idea how to play. I sit on the curb and snatch a rag out of my pocket, and I start out just wiping off all the blood and guts. Eventually, it's clean enough to play. I put my lips to the mouthpiece and blow like Satchmo. I'm playing with no training or sheet music. I'm just trying to see what's there and feel something real.

As I play, a stranger rolls up on me. They watch me fuck around for a bit and eventually they shout, "Hey buddy! Where'd you find that instrument?"

I look up from my work and think, "Who is this jabroni with no home training that's shouting me down in the street?" I'm a bit peeved, but I try not to show it. I'm still Southern, after all.

I decide to keep it cute but brief and so I simply say, "I found it inside myself." Happy to have summoned the debutante within, I go back to playing my instrument.

But the stranger is not satisfied. Head cocked, they say, "You found a whole instrument inside yourself?!"

I resist rolling my eyes.

"Yes," I reply curtly. My Cancer moon doesn't *mean* to be a bitch, but she's ready to go back to minding her business and she'd be glad to offer a demonstration of how to do so.

The stranger looks hopeful, like a puppy on adoption day. "Do you think there's an instrument inside of *me*?"

My Cancer moon sighs. How is she supposed to resist the face of a puppy on adoption day?

Shrugging off my shell of introversion, I nod Yes.

"Definitely," I tell the stranger. "I bet there's *definitely* an instrument inside of you."

So the stranger sits down next to me, and before long they've pulled out an instrument of their own. Their instrument is totally different from mine and neither of us knows how to play it, but that doesn't deter us from blowing up a storm with only our intuition as training.

As time goes by, other strangers approach and pull out their own instruments. Before you know it, we're an orchestra of novice musicians, playing tunes that none of us know. We're not playing the same songs—we're not even really trying to make music. We're just unlearning who we thought we were supposed to be.

Jessamyn has strict ideas of who she is. She's Black, fat, queer, and femme. She's an artist, a yoga teacher, a daughter, a lover, a sister, a neighbor, a scented candles advocate, a vintage furniture thrifter, an Ella Fitzgerald fan, a devotee of solitude. Jessamyn clings to the idea that her identity can always shift to accommodate an ever-evolving list of likes and dislikes.

I catch myself reciting Jessamyn's lines in my head so they sound somewhat less like bullshit when I say them out loud. I still repeat basic factoids the same way I did when I was a kid, when I was trying to memorize my birthday so I could get an Ident-A-Kid card. I test my tone for veracity, making sure the details roll off my tongue as naturally as water rolls off elephant ears.

But "Jessamyn"? She's a Mask. A Mask that conceals something more luminous and fluid than could ever be contained by epithets. Jessamyn is the case that holds my instrument. She is a vessel for what lies within and around me. The instrument inside you and me. The light that binds us together. But I get so attached to the idea of Jessamyn that I forget about the instrument inside of her. I start to confuse my Mask for the light that lives inside of me.

I never understood the weight of wearing Jessamyn, so I cling to her character description like a talisman. Without it, I fear I won't know who I am.

And I know I'm not alone because I watch my friends and family do it, too. Everyone confuses their Mask for the light and playing pretend becomes a game of survival. We get mad at ourselves when we don't perform the way we think we should, and we get mad at the people we love when they don't perform the roles we've written for them.

The week Amy Winehouse died was hot as a mother-fucker. My family was doing the all-American vacation thing in Washington, DC, where the July heat makes it feel like you're living inside of a dog's mouth. We spent our days touristing blood-stained monuments and we spent our nights shooing away mosquitos of biblical proportions. We pointed and clicked at bronze plaques, desperate for even the memory of a breeze off the Potomac. We melted in shadeless stretches of Arlington National Cemetery and huddled for shade in the shadow of Lincoln's memorial.

One night after a particularly sweaty day, my dad's Best Man came to kick it in our hotel room. Daddy's Best Man is one of those lifelong friends who always makes it feel like no time has passed even though you haven't seen him in a coon's age. Before long, Mommy, Daddy, and Daddy's Best Man were laughing over all the good times they had back when they spent their nights loitering in the parking lot of the only Hardee's in Tabor City and waiting in two-day-long lines for tickets to see the *Purple Rain* Tour.

Then, knee-deep in nostalgia with nothing to hide, Daddy's Best Man remembered how my mother had once made him the most delicious blue motorcycle he'd ever had.

Maybe finding out that your parents used to drink alcohol isn't that big of a deal to you. Maybe your parents spent your wonder years facedown in plates of pasta. But my parents were never facedown in anybody's pasta. They never mentioned alcohol at all. In fact, I was definitely a teenager before I found out the ABC store had nothing to do with alphabetizing.

Mommy looked like she'd got caught with two hands deep in the cookie jar. Her eyes darted from my brother to Daddy's Best Man to me to my father, and then, finally, resolutely, to the floor.

"I don't remember that," she told the floor.

Daddy's Best Man chuckled. "OH yOu DoN'T rEmEmBeR???" he smirked. He shrugged his shoulders and the conversation moved on.

I, however, *still* hadn't moved a muscle.

With no notice, my mother's Mask had slipped. And before she could replace it, beneath the surface of breadwinner, champion, and protector, I found myself blessed by her true luminance. Here was Tangela, freed of respectability. A light, not a bastion of morality. Someone free of definition, defying boundaries and molds. Existential and everlasting. And in the light of her truth, I was granted permission to accept my own. In my mother's truth, I saw my own.

Yoga peels back the edges of your Mask. It pushes you to the edge of who you're pretending to be, introducing you to what lies beneath. Your Mask doesn't have to distract from your luminance. In the end, it's how your light is gonna shine.

The trick is to play your own instrument, not somebody else's. Dig it out no matter the cost and play it like nobody's watching. Seek no one else's approval because the approval you seek is already inside of you. Forgive your messy corners and rough edges. You're a web of complications, and you're needed exactly as you are.

The answers to life's biggest questions are already written inside of you.

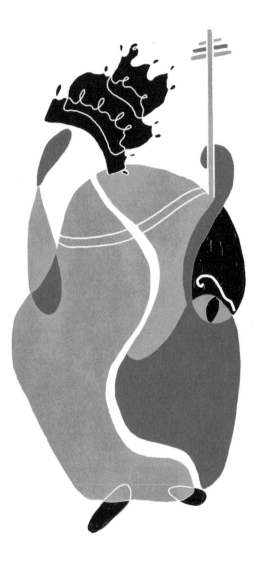

THE
HIEROPHANT

[Patanjali] "As he expounded these thoughts, his students jotted them down in a sort of shorthand using just a few words which came to be called the sutras. The literal meaning of the word sutra is 'thread'; and these sutras are just combinations of words threaded together—usually not even well-formed sentences with subjects, predicates, and so on. Within the space of these two hundred short sutras, the entire science of Yoga is clearly delineated: its aim, the necessary practices, the obstacles you may meet along the path, their removal, and precise descriptions of the results that will be obtained from such practices." (Satchidananda, 1)

"Many people simply become walking libraries . . . The Self cannot be known by theory alone . . . They usually believe you have to understand everything with the mind and that beyond it you cannot understand anything . . . How is the limited mind to understand the Unlimited One? . . . Study is all right—but not for mere logic, quoting, or fighting. Actually, it is only when you 'quote' from your own experiences that your words have weight." (Satchidananda, 78)

"Without experience we cannot understand or learn anything. Even books can only remind us of something we have experienced in the past. They help kindle a fire that is already in us." (Satchidananda, 86)

Everything that mattered to me in my childhood and adolescence was somehow connected to the Bahá'í Faith. I was born a third-generation Bahá'í in a family whose lineage has been anchored by White Christianity since before Reconstruction. Mommy's Uncle Fred was the first Bahá'í in our family. He introduced my Grandma Marvella to the Bahá'í Faith when she was pregnant with my mom. Grandma said she was hooked by the Faith from the first time she heard Fred talk about it. She knew in her gut he was speaking the truth.

Bahá'ís believe that:

- All religions pretty much say the same thing over and over again, and the essential message is do unto others as you'd have them do unto you. Each religion follows the word of what Bahá'ís call "Manifestations of God." Manifestations of God you may have heard of include Jesus, Moses, Mohammed, Buddha, and Bahá'u'lláh, the founder of the Bahá'í Faith.

- The equality of men and women functions like the wings of a dove—if one wing is broken, the bird can't fly.

- Humanity is but many waves of one ocean, and racial equality is of the utmost importance. Without racial equality, doing unto others as you'd have them do unto you isn't really a thing. Interracial marriage is highly valued, as well as open dialogue between people of varying racial identities.[2]

I imagine that ideology sounded progressive as fuck to a teen mom thugging it out in JFK's Tabor City, North Carolina, where the Ku Klux Klan is basically a political affiliation and evangelical churches remain the biggest business in town. But after Uncle Fred joined the Great Migration and moved up North, Marvella and the baby girl I call Mommy became two of Tabor City's only Bahá'ís.

Of course, when you're Black in a small southern town, church is less about religious ideology and more about having something to do on Sunday. On Sundays, my mother and grandmother, soon to be joined by my mom's younger sisters, could still be found sitting by my great-grandparents' side in the pews of Tabor City's A.M.E. Church. They may have been praise dancing in the aisles on the weekends, but Marvella and her daughters were Bahá'ís at heart.

My father was born Pentecostal on paper, but he told me he was pretty much done with church by the end of grade school. He said he'd asked his Sunday school

---

2 My grandma is sucking her teeth at me from the great beyond because she knows I'm summarizing Bahá'í ideology, and yes, there's certainly more shit I could've included here, but these are the high points and I don't have time to detail the whole of the Bahá'í Faith for you, homie.

teachers one too many questions they didn't have answers for, and that he gradually stopped taking the whole Jesus thing seriously. By the time he and Mommy got married, Daddy's apathy toward religion meant he didn't care if his kids were raised in the Bahá'í Faith. He eventually became a Bahá'í himself in the early 1990s, around the time my brother was born.

The Stanley family was involved in every aspect of the Greensboro, North Carolina, Bahá'í community, and I took every opportunity to be part of things. I only had a few friends beyond the members of The Baby-Sitters Club, so the contemporaries of my grandma who congregated around the pot of Folgers on Sunday mornings at the Bahá'í center became my BFFs.

Because the Bahá'í Faith doesn't have a clergy, within every month of the Badí' calendar there were a lot of opportunities for me to help organize shit. I could always be counted on to perform at talent nights, bring food to potlucks, collate hidden words to be read during Sunday services, or queue music for our monthly spiritual Feasts. I sang in every choir and sat faithfully at the knee of all my Sunday school teachers. I officially declared myself as a Bahá'í, a coming of age similar to confirmation or bat mitzvah, right before my fifteenth birthday, the absolute youngest age you're allowed to officially become a Bahá'í. I was basically the Bahá'í equivalent of an altar boy, minus the incense and robes. I believed my devotion to being a good Bahá'í girl was next to godliness. I thought being a good Bahá'í would make me a good person.

But beyond the virtues of parent-sanctioned volunteerism, I had little understanding of what it meant to actually *be* a Bahá'í. I memorized prayers and passages without contextualizing or comprehending what the words actually *meant*. I embodied the Hierophant, someone who clings to tradition and custom, and I thought regurgitation equaled appreciation.

I drank the Kool-Aid without asking what was in my cup. I didn't inquire as to the logic of my religious beliefs. I believed that complete obedience in my religious beliefs was my duty and responsibility. But as you might expect, it didn't take much to uproot a faith so loosely planted.

I started questioning the Bahá'í Faith shortly after I declared. I probably could've held out longer, but my hormones made the premarital celibacy required of Bahá'ís feel like a promise I might not be able to keep.

One Sunday as the millennium approached, instead of sitting front row center at the Greensboro Bahá'í Center, your girl could be found laid out on yet *another* twin bed with a boy who really couldn't have cared less about anyone's religious mores, let alone mine. His mouth was on mine, and we licked each other like pound puppies. His hands meandered from the crest of my collarbone to my belly button, but I continued to deflect his mumbled requests to finger-fuck me by reminding him that it was "against my religion." I was simultaneously appalled by his desires and deeply curious what would happen if I stepped a toe over the line of depravity. I may have kept my legs shut that day, but my days of being a good little Bahá'í girl were numbered.

Coming out queer shredded what remained of my childhood devotion to the Bahá'í faith. I've been lusting after tits and ass since childhood, but I confirmed I was "different" by middle school after developing a head-over-heels crush on my super-femme Bosnian-refugee backyard neighbor. Well, that *and* my Angelfire searches almost always dead-ended in lesbian circle jerks. I tried my best to ignore it, but by the time I got to high school, it was pretty clear that I was a total gaymo.

Coming out to my BFFs wasn't the issue. It was coming out to my parents that had me buggin'.

Before breaking the news, I did some exploratory research into how the Bahá'í Faith feels about homosexuality. I'd never had reason to research it in the past because I really didn't know any gay people, plus I hadn't spent much time actually thinking about my sexuality. My surrogate godfather is gay as the day is long, but we never really openly talked about his sexuality. He and his partner were just there, in the background of our family life, without any explanatory parentheticals. Frankly, I kinda hoped I might outgrow my lesbian proclivities. I mean, I'd outgrown children's clothing sizes and my baby teeth, so why not outgrow my hormones?

I was devastated to find that while the Bahá'í writings expound the progressive virtues of racial equality and emphasize the importance of interracial relationships, the Bahá'í Faith still somehow managed to be low-key homophobic. The discrimination may have been coded, but I'm Southern and we are well versed at reading between the lines of bigotry. I found lines in Bahá'í sacred texts comparing homosexuals to leprosy patients. Just like leprosy, homosexuality was considered to be a contagious disease. It's not like Bahá'ís were encouraged to commit hate crimes or any shit like that, but we *were* encouraged to stay as far from homosexuality as possible for fear of catching an infectious disease.[3]

So . . . I'd say that's *not* a great thing to read if you're worried about your religious family disowning you. It certainly didn't instill a lot of faith that my parents would be cool with my sexuality, and like many a closet case before me, I resolved to conceal the truth for as long as possible.

But "as long as possible" had an expiration date. My lie by omission got to be *so* big—too big to fit in anybody's closet. When I finally broke the news, Mommy sobbed and said she wasn't sure what to do with the information, which sounded like Mom-speak for not knowing how to tell her friends she'd accidentally given

---

3 It's true that the twenty-first century has yielded a progressive shift in Bahá'í moral standards, but back when ya girl was coming out of the closet, the Bahá'í Faith was not down with the gay agenda.

birth to a dyke. Daddy just seemed glad that my surprise revelation was homosexuality and not unplanned pregnancy, but he's always been a pragmatist that way.

But once the dust settled, neither of my parents wanted to talk about it. They both pretended like nothing happened, and since they also gave birth to a Cancer sun, I followed suit. For years, we never talked about my sexuality. I think they hoped that coming out to your parents was a mid-aughts trend that might go out of style if they ignored it.

But it turned out that the only thing I outgrew was feeling like I had shit to hide. I grew tired of being ashamed of my identity. By my early twenties, I was both out of the closet and fully untethered from the Bahá'í Faith.

Sacred texts had a very strict definition when I was a kid. Mostly I just thought they had to be old, religious, and cosigned by my mom. Shit like the Kitáb-i-Aqdas and *The Hidden Words of Bahá'u'lláh* were both sanctioned. The Bible was kinda iffy—especially if King James had anything to do with it.

But when I wandered from religion in my late teens, I lost my definition of sacred texts entirely. It's only in adulthood that I've reclaimed the idea of defining my own sacred texts. My personal list includes the writings of James Baldwin, Malcolm X, Gary Zukav, Don Miguel

Ruiz, Henry David Thoreau, Swami Vivekananda, and Dr. Maya Angelou, among many others.

I consider Swami Satchidananda's translation of *The Yoga Sutras of Patanjali* to be one of my primary sacred texts, and excerpts from this text open every essay in this book. *The Yoga Sutras of Patanjali* is a body of 196 Sanskrit aphorisms about yoga practice, and it's widely considered one of the foundational texts of American yoga, though not all schools of yoga hold it in such esteem. The sutras have been passed down for thousands of years and translated an untold number of times.

Even though it was a required text of my yoga teacher training, I've gotta tell you that I breezed through the sutras during YTT like a grade-schooler shovels down their summer reading on the last night of vacation. If SparkNotes had been available, a bitch would have gladly read those instead.

To say I didn't care about *The Yoga Sutras of Patanjali* would be an overstatement of their importance in my life. The first time I read them for context was at least a year after my 200-hour YTT, and it felt a lot like reading my own journal but written in someone else's handwriting. The aphorisms hit me in the chest like an edict from the universe.

Since then, I've read and listened to several translations of Patanjali's sutras, but I feel a particular kinship with Swami Satchidananda's translation and commentary. Swami Satchidananda was a prolific Indian spiritual teacher who taught around the world until his death in the early aughts. He founded the Integral Yoga Institute in New York City and Yogaville in Buckingham, Virginia, and served as opening speaker of the Woodstock Music and Arts Festival in 1969.

Satchidananda made a lot of observations about the human condition that feel *very* fucking familiar to me. When I'm reading his words, it's like we're kicking it on the couch with a blunt, mulling over the meaning of life. We don't always agree. Satchidananda's translations of the sutras piss me off sometimes. There are spots where I've gesticulated wildly with my fork in simultaneous agreement and disagreement, shaking my head yes while nodding my head no. But his statements about the spiritual essence of the universe always bring tears to my eyes because they are both very complex and so simple. His words are his Truth, and his Truth is my Truth. I see myself in his stories. His commentary reads like prayer to me.

And yet. I don't think I need to hang on to any sacred texts for dear life. Even Swami Satchidananda didn't think it was a great idea to fret over sacred texts. He said, "Use it and pass it on." There's nothing you can learn from another person that you couldn't understand more clearly from within yourself. Your truest connection with the god of your own understanding happens inside yourself, not with someone else.

What sacred texts *can* do is provide context for the Truth that is always living inside you. Maybe you've got access to your Truth but the words are slightly out of focus and the characters are unfamiliar. The words of others can help translate a Truth that might otherwise be impossible to comprehend.

The sutras and passages woven through this book may have helped me figure out some shit, but I've gotta remind myself not to get too caught up in them. They're just words, after all. Swami Satchidananda's *Yoga Sutras of Patanjali* is just one man's translation of a very old text. A very old text that was once nothing more than the thoughts of a teacher whose students diligently recorded what he said. *The Yoga Sutras of Patanjali* offers a road map for discovering a manifesto that's already written inside you. The only reason the sutras make any sense is because they speak the language of the soul. The book itself isn't nearly as important as the Truth it expresses, which is both timeless and crucial. Take the message and leave the text behind. Pass it on to someone else. Retreat within it for the solace and companionship offered by the sentiments, but don't overly identify with the pages themselves.

The Fast is a period of spiritual cleansing before Naw Ruz, the Bahá'í New Year. Every year, during the nineteen days before the vernal equinox, Bahá'ís abstain from eating and drinking from dawn till dusk.

Every year after turning my back on the Bahá'í Faith, I continued to participate in the Fast. But I fasted out of habit, not because I understood its merit.

As a child of American consumer capitalism, I often have difficulty telling the difference between my needs and wants. I guess that's what happens when an agrarian society matures into industrialized life. You end up with generations of consumers who are bloated by choice, believing they deserve everything their hearts desire and who ignore the connection between body, mind, and spirit.

Fasting is a common practice in most religions because it escorts you to spiritual destinations otherwise hard to come by. Not to be confused with disordered eating, intentional abstinence from food and water is spiritually invigorating. It requires digging beneath the surface of choice to experience something more. It means fortifying yourself from the inside, instead of expecting fortification from the outside world.

But mindset is crucial. Fasting out of obligation is *so* different from fasting out of spiritual necessity. I've been fasting for almost twenty years and it took at least a decade of those years to understand any of this philosophical shit.

I don't know about you, but much of my day is anchored by eating and drinking. Making plans for food and drink takes up a considerable amount of my consciousness. Sometimes I think I need to eat, but upon closer inspection, I'm just bored or lonely. But it's only when I abstain from eating altogether that I can tell the difference.

More than anything else, fasting is a ritual that takes me beyond myself, without filter or adulteration.

The first few hours of fasting are relatively easy to bear. Before sunrise I wake up, say my prayers, practice yoga postures, meditate, and eat a little breakfast. Mostly I try to drink as much water as possible. By lunchtime I'm not usually all that hungry, so I intentionally focus on other things—a work project, perhaps.

For me, the hardest part of the day is usually sometime between 3 p.m. and 6 p.m. That's when the shit hits the fan and the rubber meets the road. Those are the hours right before I usually break the fast, and what happens during that time is what the fuss is all about. It's not like I'm dying of hunger or even feeling woozy—I'm sure it felt like that when I was a kid, but what doesn't feel unbearable at that age?

No, it's more like the average drudgery of my life, shit that typically wouldn't make me raise an eyebrow, becomes a nonstop mind fuck. I start to doubt myself and I think ill of my intentions. I talk cash shit about myself. It's not unlike practicing yoga postures. There's always a moment in yoga's physical practice when your mind and your ego start to fuck with your resolve. And by the time your ego kicks into gear, it doesn't matter how strong you felt when shit got started.

Likewise, no matter how much water I drank at the start of the day or how hungry I *wasn't* at lunchtime, there comes a point in every fasting day when I contemplate sucking dick for a tug on a stranger's CamelBak.

Fasting becomes an exploration of what it actually means to be thirsty and hungry. To exist without and beyond. Thirst and hunger drag me kicking and screaming to the present moment, much like yoga. To experience need and to experience my behavior *when* I need. To observe my thoughts without judgment and anger. That mind fuck is what fasting is all about. Fasting draws a line between bullshit and truth to make space for what really matters. It opens up contemplation and introspection that'd be otherwise impossible.

It's pretty poetic, then, that my 200-hour yoga teacher training fell squarely at the start of the Fast and when I realized that the dates were gonna line up, I considered skipping it altogether that year.

As much as I respect the practice of fasting, it seemed vaguely ludicrous to abstain from both food *and* water during a physically arduous yoga teacher training that was pretty much guaranteed to kick my ass. But the more I thought about not fasting, the more I began to question why I was looking for a way to get out of it. I thought of all the times in high school and college that I'd sought any excuse under the sun to get out of fasting, even getting wasted all night and sleeping all day to ward off the desire to eat while the sun was up.

Instead of finding yet another cop-out, I surprised myself by committing to the fast during YTT. I told myself not to make too big a deal of it and gave myself permission to stop at any point.

Every day during training, instead of congregating with my fellow trainees over sandwiches and salads, I'd retreat into solitude. I spent a lot of time alone, in silence, smoking weed, and pondering life.

Sometimes yoga people liken our practices to assembling an internal fire. The Sanskrit word for internal fire is *tapas*, and I always think of tapas as the fire that burns away the pieces of ourselves that don't need to be there. Every time we link breath and physical movement, it's like throwing kindling on our internal campfire. During my YTT, fasting bellowed the flames of my fire. It showed me how much of a whiny little bitch I can be, how self-righteous I am, and how much I adore projecting those emotions onto other people.

That was the year fasting stopped feeling like a performance. Instead, it became about laying myself bare and cleansing myself from the inside out. It elevated my yoga from a glorified exercise program to a restorative practice of Self. It also provided a path toward acceptance of yogic spirituality, which is accessible to practitioners of every religious faith. Yogic spirituality speaks to the soul's eternal condition, beyond religious systems, rhetoric, and culture.

But fasting isn't really about religion, either. Or rather, it's not about religion beyond the religion of self-acceptance. That's really my religion. My church is the church of self-acceptance and every body is welcome at the altar. Even if it doesn't feel like it, all roads always lead to self-acceptance.

As soon as I'm ready, I can let go of the good little Bahá'í girl act. But that doesn't mean I have to turn away from Faith. Religion is temporal and the spirit of God is much bigger than any man's religion. I don't have to be held hostage by what I disagree with in the Bahá'í Faith.

Both the Bahá'í Faith and yoga are just ideologies and I'm only held by them if I want to be. Ideology isn't the answer, it's just the beginning of another question.

Yoga showed me how to reconcile with the Bahá'í Faith and accept the homophobia in Bahá'í writings as a reflection of the cultural context in which they were born. I don't have to define myself solely through the lens of what it *looks* like to be a Bahá'í. I don't have to pretend to be something I'm not. If I want to fast, I can fast. I can read the writings, ponder their relevance in my life, and let them go. Just like any other sacred text.

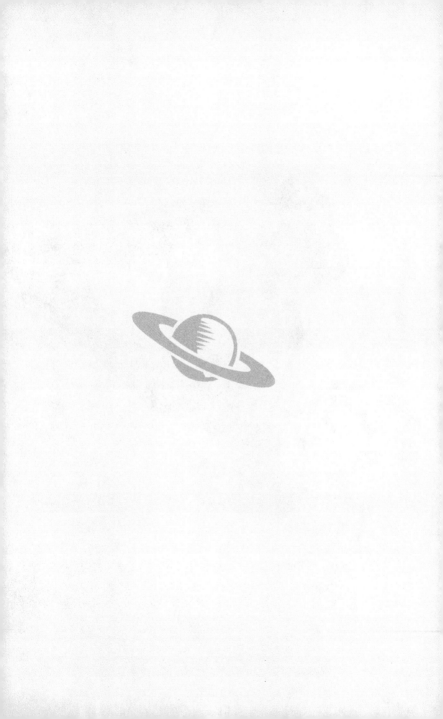

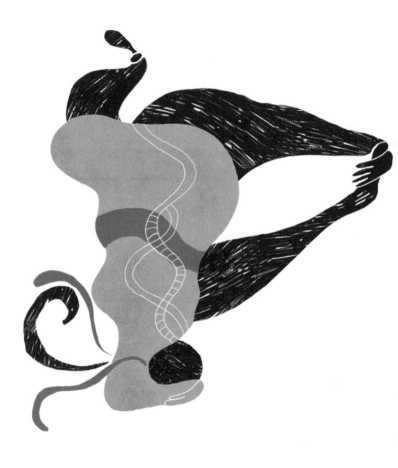

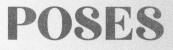

POSES

"Asana means the posture that brings comfort and steadiness. Any pose that brings this comfort and steadiness is an asana. If you can achieve one pose, that is enough . . . Unless the body is perfectly healthy and free from all toxins and tensions, a comfortable pose is not easily obtained . . . The body must be so supple it can bend any way you want it to." (Satchidananda, 143)

"If the body is still, it is easy to make the mind still . . . If we sit that long, the mind comes under our control automatically. Through the body we can put a brake on the mind . . . If we decide, 'I'm not moving for three hours,' the mind ultimately has to obey us, because it needs the body's cooperation in order to get anything. That is the benefit of asana siddhi, or accomplishment of asana." (Satchidananda, 145)

"Even a cloth must undergo tapas to become clean . . . The mind too must be washed, squeezed, tossed, dried, and ironed. Don't think that if someone causes us pain they hate us, but rather that they are helping us to purify ourselves . . . If we understand this point and accept it, we'll never find fault with anybody who abuses, scolds, or insults us." (Satchidananda, 138–39) hen I started practicing yoga, I really didn't give a fuck about anything but the poses. All this yogic philosophy I've been jabbering about? Man, that shit didn't make any sense to me. Honestly, I wasn't even sure if I was *allowed* to care because back then, I really wasn't sure whether people who aren't Indian should even be practicing yoga at all.

When you hear the word *yoga*, it's almost always defined as a physical exercise. Classical yoga teachers have always extolled the virtues of yogic spirituality, but postures are still the primary language of American yoga.

Postures are a great introduction to the basics of yoga practice, but they're not meant to serve as your sole path to inner knowledge. They're just a great way to get children prepped for meditation. Vinyasa-style yoga classes were actually developed as energy maintenance for children, particularly young boys.

You're always a child in the infancy of your yoga journey, no matter how old you are when you first step onto the mat. The postures are an introduction to the core elements of a spirituality beyond religiosity. Sometimes, simply moving the body and connecting to the breath are all you need to set foot on the path toward transcendence.

I think the poses are easy for Americans to understand because they fit into our worldview. Americans value physical beauty over almost anything else—and therefore we value dedication to physical refinement.

Postural work is a familiar recitation of the same narrative we've been fed since birth. A narrative wherein physical health is the ultimate wealth, and the decay of the physical body marks the end of all that matters.

But what's the real purpose of keeping your body in perfect condition? To prevent it from aging? To keep it frozen in time? But the art of aging is life's great crescendo. Your aging is your loudest moment, your greatest depth. You exist to age. I think the art of aging is to age with humility and grace. To age and enjoy the process. To welcome age with open arms. Obsessing over the human body's physical condition and postures is another way of trying not to age.

Poses don't really matter that much, but according to the yoga industrial complex, a strong yoga practice means you have to be able to turn your spine inside out like Linda Blair in *The Exorcist* while holding a handstand on the edge of a mountain. General wisdom says that the more poses you know, the better you are at yoga, and the better you are at yoga, the better you are at being alive. That being able to contort your body means you're a good person, maybe even a better person than somebody else. But is that what yoga's about? Being a better person than somebody else?

Not hardly. How can you be a better person than somebody else? That's not a thing. And that's precisely the spot where the yoga industrial complex fucked up the game. Because yoga isn't ever about trying to get one up on anybody. That's supremacy you're thinking of. Supremacy is all about being better and having more than those around you.

Capitalism is the child of supremacy, and capitalism is pretty much the only reason that many of us, myself included, have ever even heard of yoga. But yoga was here way before capitalism was the loudest voice in the room, and it exists beyond what capitalism can define. And no matter how many poses you practice, whether you're upside down or inside out or twisted into a pretzel, you'll always end up drawing that exact same conclusion. That there's no amount of yoga postures that will make you better than anybody else.

Ultimately, mastering postures is a moot point. Postures aren't about getting shit perfect. After all, you were already perfect before the postures, and being able to practice them isn't gonna shift that truth.

I think obsessively practicing yoga postures, especially drilling the same ones over and over again, is a lot like scratching an itch or picking at a scab. If I'm being honest, I know that I've used postures as a form of self-mutilation. I've drilled sun salutations and repetitively practiced deep back bends and inversions for the same reasons that I have been known to chew my cuticles until the beds are stained with blood. Because it feels good to hurt myself.

I wanted to hold on to the headstands and splits and wheels because they felt like proof that I once knew the Truth. I covet the photos of my practice like they're Girl Scout badges, like they're gold stars adhered to my forehead before lunch. Look, Mama, today in school I learned how to achieve bliss. I learned how to be okay. I learned how to live. I learned how to do it right.

No matter how toned your abs get, some kind of spiritual reckoning is always on your horizon. Postures exhaust your physical body so your mind can arrive in the present moment. When a yoga pose kicks the shit out of your physical body, the mind is (finally) able to rest. When the muscles, bones, and ligaments work together, it's like plugging into the truth of all that Is, and only when your whole body is integrated is it possible to see within yourself. But the yogic path is just preparation for Death, the final stage in your inevitable decay. It's not a preventive measure, but it's a way of showing up fully for both the voyage and the destination of the infinite.

Gradually, for one reason or another, your body is gonna stop working the way it once did. And as your skin wrinkles and sags, you'll be forced to reckon with what lies underneath it all. And the wisdom you've gained from that inevitable reckoning will always trump the naive glory of your physicality.

Your postural work doesn't need to be particularly complicated. Honestly, you really only need to know one pose and it's called sitting the fuck down. In fact, give it a shot right now. Sit down and be quiet. You don't need to cross your legs because you don't need legs. You don't need to sit upright because lying on your back is just as legit. Are you comfortable yet? Great. Now, just try to maintain this posture.

Is your mind racing? Are you holding your breath? Are you fidgeting? Are you holding back the urge to speak? Are you worried about yesterday? Are you thinking about what's on your plate for later today?

Probably. That's chill. After all, you're human and all of that shit's totally normal. Don't try to freeze time. Just try to be here now. Just try to bear witness to yourself.

Breathing your way into the present moment is the whole function of yoga postures. The single purpose of every posture is to bear witness to your fidgets and your held breaths and the cacophony of noise echoing in your mind. And in my experience, trying to do all this shit in a shape like criss-cross applesauce is hard enough without also mimicking a Cirque du Soleil contortionist.

But just because poses aren't the most important part of yoga doesn't mean they're not still lit. When you focus on your body, you situate yourself in the present moment. There's nowhere else to turn toward but right now. Working on your postures is beautiful and it offers so many lessons. Postural work is like a really good metaphor, and like a really good metaphor, every posture is so much more than it seems on the surface.

In every pose, whether you're right side up or upside down, revel in the magnitude of what it is to experience your full attention. From that space, give yourself permission to focus entirely on how your body behaves. Explore how every single piece of your meat suit arrives in this exact moment. In every pose, consider how your head is hanging and in what direction your heart is beating. Consider that if you breathe more intentionally, it may even be possible to relax that tiny sliver of muscle right between your butt cheeks. Consider the tension held between your eyebrows and between the wrinkles in your knees. Enjoy the curious sensation as your jaw finally unhinges.

Consider all of this and more in every posture, from easy pose to scorpion handstand. The shape of the posture or how long you hold it or whether or not you use props is irrelevant. And maybe this doesn't need to be said but I'm still gonna say it: What anyone else has to say about what your body looks like in the posture is *especially* irrelevant.

I really can't overemphasize this point. You know as well as I do that your body is gonna keep changing every day for the rest of your life. Your body literally feels different every day and I agree that the constant change is pretty obnoxious. There's always some new ache or pang or a hair that wasn't there before or some cancer that wasn't there before or whatever bullshit card that life's petty bitch ass has decided to slide your way. You can really count on the wheel of fortune to always keep turning no matter what, and luck won't always be on your side. Regardless of your age, or the time of day, or how long it's been since your last meal, no matter what's going on in your body. No matter how you look today. No matter who you *are* today.

By moving your body, you can find some version of stillness. And actually, what we call stillness is really just the energetic space between inhales and exhales of motion. What looks like stillness is really just the same science that makes zoetropes so magical.

Since stillness is found in motion, I like to put my body in motion to find it. Not always, but definitely sometimes. I find that I can only *really* be still once I've moved my body around, sometimes a little and sometimes a whole fucking lot. Especially if I've spent a lot of time plugged into the matrix. If I've been caught up in work or if my Mask is on too tight, it can be helpful to jostle my body a little to get my mind pointing in the right direction. Intitially, that process can feel fucking brutal depending on what I had for breakfast or when I fell asleep or who has pissed me off most recently or how long it's been since I've had a moment alone. Depending on all these factors and more, my body might not be interested in stillness because it's congested with everything I've ingested and digested, physically, mentally, and emotionally.

Postural flows don't have to be complicated on paper. You don't have to practice three firefly poses in a row to get beneath the surface of your Self. I don't know, I say that and then I think that some people obviously really *do* need that. They *do* need to practice three firefly poses in a row to be still. In fact, it stands to reason that if you're a really physically active person, you may need to keep upping the ante as your body acclimates to a high intensity interval postural style in order to arrive at stillness.

But that withstanding, sometimes the most basic shit is all you really need. And sometimes poses that seem really simple end up being harder than anything else.

I think the hardest part of practicing poses is mental rather than physical. The lessons they provoke are oceanic mind fucks, pulling up shit I'd rather ignore, sometimes stuff I've been ignoring on purpose for decades. Crying is a regular state of affairs and within the solitude of the postures, there's all the time in the world to cry like a little baby.

The hardest poses usually offer the best lessons. They taste like Robitussin on the way down, but they'll clear out your spiritual congestion like none other. There's a beauty to the difficulty and an elegance to the pain— really, the complexity of them is decadent. The pain and the difficulty have so much to teach, and leaving them out is like spoiling the punchline of a really great joke.

In my experience, the poses are always pulling up some shit you've needed to deal with for years, maybe even since you were born. But even though it always feels good to let your wounds breathe, that don't make it smell any better when you peel back the bandage.

For me, it's twisting postures. They're a mind fuck for me. I've historically hated them because they make me work my gut and working toward better gut health has turned into an unexpected journey of my post–Saturn Return. Which is to say I know *way* more about enzymes and probiotics now than I did before my twenty-seventh birthday. But I digress.

Twisting postures are particularly good for the gut because they wring out the organs in your midsection. Twisting your midsection is really the only way that a lot of your bodily organs will ever get massaged. Liver, stomach, pancreas, small intestine, large intestine—all of that shit. Twisting massages your organs and when they're massaged, they can work at optimal capacity.

But if you're like me and you don't twist your midregion that much, your organs can't get massaged. And when they don't get a little massage every now and then, they don't work that well. Just like your shoulders and lower back, every part of your physical body needs to be massaged from time to time.

But for a bitch like me, twisting postures don't always feel that great. Sometimes, they can feel downright terrible, like catshit spread on a cracker. I find twists that some people consider basic to be complicated as fuck. Sometimes they even feel painful.

Here's what I do. When the postures start to feel painful, I back the fuck off. And there's a striking difference between sensation and pain—I could try to explain it, but I won't because it's really something you have to understand for yourself. But once you understand the difference, it becomes a lot easier to make even the most physically challenging postures accessible for where your body is today, not where it could be in the future or where it once was in the past.

I spend much of my postural practice figuring out ways to make the poses feel more accessible for my body as it is right now, not how it was yesterday or how it might be tomorrow. Not necessarily more comfortable, but certainly more bearable.

Once I find a way to practice a posture that's most accessible to how my body feels today, I'm able to just try breathing in that posture for as long as possible. As my breath develops, my posture deepens. As for breathing, that's a whole other kettle of fish entirely, but suffice it to say: Breathing is a lot more complicated than settling on and into anybody's yoga posture.

Whether or not you start practicing yoga solely for the physical benefits is irrelevant. If you commit to the path of yoga, you'll always end up seeing yourself. It's no accident that most yoga postures mimic the kinesiology of other creatures, both mortal and mythological. I think it's easier to connect with my body when I'm embodying the attributes of other creatures. I'm present to my subtle body, my unseen body, my full spiritual self that encompasses everything that lives and breathes, in both this world and what lies beyond.

The subtle, spiritual body guides all yoga practice. The physical body grows frail with time, but the subtle body grows more virile and wise with every passing day.

Being good at yoga poses won't make you immortal. Short of coming upon a vampire in a dark alley, immortality probably ain't gon' be a thing for most of us. Every superpower you seek is already happening inside of you. If it's immortality you seek, you might do better to spend a little less time thinking about yoga and more time hanging out at Fangtasia. You might end up as somebody's dinner, but it's a better path to immortality than postural mastery.

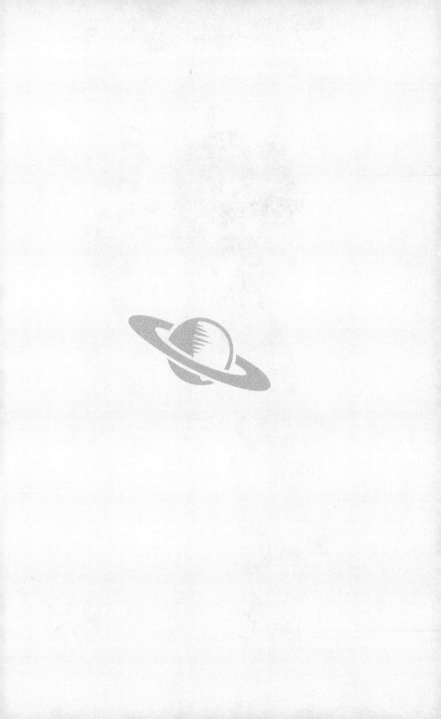

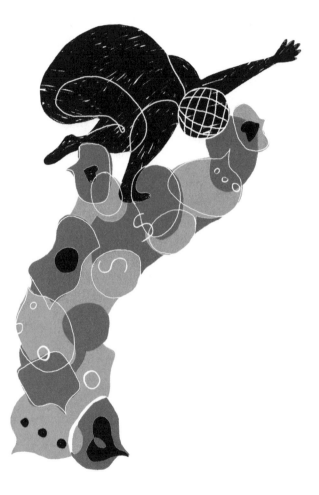

WEALTH
& OTHER
AMERICAN VALUES

4.4 - "A yogi's ego sense alone is the cause of [other] artificially created minds." (Satchidananda, 199)

"'If my disciples leave me one after another, what will happen to me?'" (Satchidananda, 94)

"If they come to you, let them come; enjoy their presence. But when they go, enjoy their departure, too . . . In reality, nothing is bad in this world . . . Real pleasure comes from detaching ourselves completely from the entire world, in standing aloof—making use of the world as a master of it. Only in that can we have pride . . . Wherever we go, the world follows." (Satchidananda, 95)

1.26 - "Unconditioned by time, Isvara[4] is the teacher of even the most ancient teachers." (Satchidananda, 38)

---

4 Isvara—the supreme cosmic soul; God (Satchidananda, 228).

A few years ago, a family friend asked if he could use my yoga career as the subject of his film school thesis. If I'm being honest, the whole thing was embarassing and I did all I could to put the kibosh on it before it got too serious, but the jig was up when the aforementioned family friend got my mom involved. My mother is a polite Southern Belle and no daughter of hers was gonna deny a family friend a few harmless interview sessions.

Up until that point, my mom had mostly ignored that I made a living out of hustling yoga classes, aside from wondering how this decision would ever square with paying off my student loans. In spite of her skepticism, both she and my father seemed very excited by the prospect of being profiled alongside me in the film. In their interview, my parents went on and on about how they felt that my work as a yoga teacher was a clear extension of my adolescent musical theater obsession. They drew a direct and succinct line between my yoga teaching practice and a teenhood spent in a near-constant reenactment of *A Chorus Line* and *Cats*, sometimes performing them concurrently. Suddenly, it made total sense that Mommy was ignoring my work. It was as natural as tuning out my umpteenth rendition of "Dance Ten, Looks Three" warbling up from the trunk of her '88 Oldsmobile station wagon.

I was horribly embarrassed that my parents would make my yoga practice sound like New Age vaudeville, but where was the lie? Singing and dancing *was* one of the first ways I received affection.

Practicing yoga has never felt like a performance to me. In fact, learning to play the instrument inside of me is how I stop performing. When I'm practicing yoga, I feel like I'm finally living off script.

But teaching American yoga, especially in the age of social media, *is* a performance. Teaching American yoga is more like being a chorus girl than anything else. That's why so many of us yoga teachers are former or current performers.

Instead of learning to play spiritual instruments, teaching American yoga has a lot more to do with convincing other people to attend your yoga classes and trying to get them to like you. As a result, I've always resented being a yoga teacher. It's all vocal warm-ups and remembering to cheat out and "Sing out, Louise!" It's only because I spent my adolescence pretending to be Judy Garland that I've ever been able to hack it as a professional American yoga teacher.

It's really not a coincidence that the yoga industrial complex measures success by the same metrics that govern Hollywood. You can see traces of celebrity culture idolatry in everything I do. YouTube has been my church, and I've bowed before the altar of Instagram.

At this point, it doesn't even matter if I *want* to perform because people show up expecting to see what social media's advertised. Their class registration has strings attached. It's our shared covenant. Mats unfurled and legs crossed, they expect a show, whether I feel like giving one or not.

If you're doing it right, practicing yoga is where performance goes to die. But it's hard to tell the difference between practicing yoga and a *Star Search* audition when you've programmed yourself to shuffle ball change.

We think the best yoga teachers have packed classes the same way we always think the best restaurant is the one with a line around the block and the best sweater is the one that's out of stock. Perception of American yogic teaching ability always comes down to class attendance and whether or not you have a full waitlist. Social media has become the audition, and waiting for your class to fill is like waiting for the cast list to go up. It feels like your path to enlightenment will only come by way of meteoric follower accumulation.

Every prominent American yoga lineage has been impacted by celebrity culture, even as far back as Swami Vivekananda and his nineteenth-century lectures at the World's Parliament of Religions. Much of B. K. S. Iyengar's American yoga success was the result of his ability to sell the yoga lifestyle to wealthy Americans. Mainstream spirituality has pretty much always relied upon celebrity culture, even if it's just the celebrity culture of the NextDoor app. Hoes always wanna find a way to remember their spirit and keep up with the Joneses at the same time. Jivamukti, Bikram, Y7—they all benefit from celebrity culture.

In the financial transaction between American yoga teachers and their students, spiritual awareness becomes a commodity. The yoga industrial complex relies upon wealthy people believing that spirituality is a material resource controlled by yoga teachers, who are expected to be deified. These teachers, who are spiritual seekers just like the students they serve, are cast in the role of demigod. The student believes they are paying for both the teacher's wisdom and a guarantee of gradually becoming the teacher's spiritual equal. Basically, the student and the teacher will eventually get to be demigods together! The American yoga practitioner is expected to enjoy singing capitalism's siren song. In my experience, this is the relationship that an American yoga teacher must accept in order to climb the ladder of success.

Humans are always seeking power, and yoga becomes yet another way to accumulate it. It might be power over your children or lovers or coworkers. It might be power over your neighbors. It might be power over your hairdresser. It might be power over strangers, people you know only through your computer screen. You seek power because you seek recognition. You crave recognition because you want someone, anyone, to tell you that you're doing a good job of pretending to be the person you've decided to become, and that the mask has come to fit your face. You want confirmation that you're doing it right. But the confirmation you seek can only be found inside yourself.

Yoga is the reminder that everything you seek is already happening inside of you all the time. But what about yoga in the era when everyone, even your great-grandma, is looking for validation on the internet? When followers become proof of life, proof of identity, proof of purpose?

The quest for followers trips me up every time. Hubris and greed are my shadow side, and seeking followers never fails to dilute my message while also distancing me from my mission. I surely sought the limelight, but a bitch definitely didn't know what she was getting herself into. I didn't understand the damage caused by standing in artificial light. A light that beams from others is subject to fluctuations in both luster and opacity. I underestimated what it feels like to bask in a beam of liquid gold one minute and have it snuffed into obsidian without notice.

Consumerism is America's religion, but it's an unsatisfactory replacement for spiritual practice. Spiritual dissatisfaction is at the core of our collective unhappiness. Capitalism thrives when you hate yourself and there'll always be a cuter dress, a more impressive house, or a better pair of shoes. Nothing you buy will ever be enough, and it's set up that way by design. But while capitalism is all about looking outside your Self, yoga says the exact opposite. Yoga and capitalism are like oil and water: They just don't go together.

In my experience, American yoga culture has less to do with spiritual comprehension and more to do with buying shit. Acquiring possessions has become the primary metric of spiritual comprehension. But that tracks with the rest of American society. Americans value performance of life over embodied living. We cling to our masks and idolize celebrity culture. We live our lives like vaguely scripted reality shows. But when we inevitably realize just how little can be gained from worshipping money, the vast darkness that follows can be fatally debilitating. Capitalism provides no context for the afterlife, so we walk around unaware of our ever-present divinity.

Since wealth is the American religion, we don't question consumerism's presence in the yoga world. But maybe it *should* be questioned. Every yoga person eventually realizes that money plus power will never equal bliss. Personally, I think the wealth that usually accompanies American yoga practitioners shows that wealthy people are more aware of this than anyone else. I've often wondered if children born of wealth are quickest to embrace yoga because they're exposed to capitalism's empty promises straight out of the gate.

Capitalism offers no concept of spirituality—just wealth acquisition and idolatry. The intersection of capitalism and yoga is particularly gruesome. Yoga teachers perform as jesters in the courts of their students. And how, I ask, are you supposed to provide a spiritual mirror for your fellow practitioners if you're trying to figure out how to lick their assholes at the same time? I can tell you from personal experience that it's a weird angle from which to see yourself reflected.

It's a certain type of person who becomes an American yoga teacher, especially in the digital age. Becoming a licensed, insurance-card-carrying yoga teacher requires enough liquid capital to pay for yoga teacher training and all the associated accoutrements. It requires excess time and energy to both practice and contemplate the esoteric. For a long time, rich White people were the only ones who fit this equation, but as time has progressed, so has the diversity of American yoga teachers.

The first lesson of teaching yoga in the digital age is don't suck dick for free because you'll end up broke with chapped lips. Every corner of capitalism has a price, and it's better to know yours than to pretend the limit does not exist. But I've gotta tell you—I can't speak for anyone else, but I need to find a separation between yoga and money because the combination is polluting my soul. I think money and spirituality are generally a problematic combo. Money distorts the communion between fellow seekers by festering socioeconomic hierarchies. All human beings are grown from the same soil, regardless of how much money we've got. None among us has a monopoly on spiritual connection to the divine, and wealth won't bridge the divide to enlightenment any faster than poverty.

Much of the American yoga industrial complex consists of us selling iterations of the practice to each other as a means of supporting our personal capitalist agendas. On one hand, maybe this is the literal antithesis of yoga, but on the other hand it's created a very interesting sociological experiment. Instead of nomadically retreating from the confines of capitalist society, American yoga practitioners find ways to finance the pursuit of spiritual truth while still swimming in the mainstream.

American yoga practitioners expect to pay for their yoga in the same way they expect to pay for everything else. In return, I expect to sing for my supper. But my heart's not in the show anymore. At best, teaching yoga is an offering of self-reflection to others. Charging money for the privilege of self-reflection makes me feel gross. I always end up behaving like a good little capitalist and charging for my services. Bitches gotta eat, after all, and so does my team. But it still makes me feel gross.

Teaching yoga on social media means fighting with your ego every day. Praying that it doesn't eventually swell so large that you turn into a blimp. It means checking, constantly checking. It means posting, constantly posting. It means creating, constantly creating. But always with the other person in mind, always with your followership riding shotgun. The follower begins to color your inner sight. It becomes hard to see yourself without them. It's hard to know yourself without them. It means constantly thinking of ways to do better, to do more than the other guy. It's a never-ending state of comparison—no amount of work is ever enough and the idea of "good enough" becomes a fantastical myth. I don't think it's possible to work in social media without these feelings eventually rising to the surface. Frankly, I don't think you can engage with social media at *all* without eventually arriving on this page.

But cave drawings and hieroglyphics were the original social media feed. And if Instagram had existed in pre-Partition India, B. K. S. Iyengar would've been the OG IG kid. Social media is an evolution of the show-and-telling that has pretty much always been a staple of human behavior. In social media, I'm embedded in the world of my people. Me and my people are obsessed with what we look like. We feed off the adoration of others. We look outside ourselves for the home that already exists within. We tranquilize and intoxicate ourselves to dull what it feels like to be alive. We're taking the edge off our constant repetition of lies and conflation. Our digital avatars become yet another mask atop our light. Me and my people are strangers to ourselves. In response, our children are absorbing this behavior, and now their self-worth is irrevocably tied to the impact of social media.

I'm always reminding myself to question the internet, question social media, question the art of curating my avatar at the expense of understanding my actual identity. We're in a digital war, and the mind is its battlefield. I think I expect my avatar to somehow be a better version of myself. I expect her to be better than the me I embody in real life. Against my better judgment, I respect royalty and expect hierarchy. I expect to be represented by who I hope to be rather than who I know myself to be, and I admire the avatars of those who pretend to be what feels just out of my reach, rather than what lives beneath my surface.

I think the internet has dramatically evolved how spiritual rhetoric will be conveyed, just like how the written word changed and evolved spiritual discourse. Everything changed when bitches got access to pen and paper. What had previously only been conveyed orally could suddenly be spread and shared with the masses. But I think mystics and skeptics of earlier generations would've needed to write fewer books if they'd had access to the internet. Fuck the number of people that can read your book. Think of how many people can casually engage with your Instagram posts. It becomes possible to influence an entire generation before breakfast with the same energy you're using to take a shit.

It's true that sometimes yoga can become solely about followership but, if I'm being honest, I think that's probably fine. I think every version of the practice is probably fine, because the message always ends up being the same. The destination is always the same. Vapid as it is, tap dancing for Instagram likes still got me to self-acceptance. Social media provides an accurate, shocking, and embarrassing mirror in which to view my truth, and by standing on my internet soapbox, people I will never meet are invited to view their truth as well. It may seem like the digital age trivializes yoga, but is the spread of compassion ever *really* trivial?

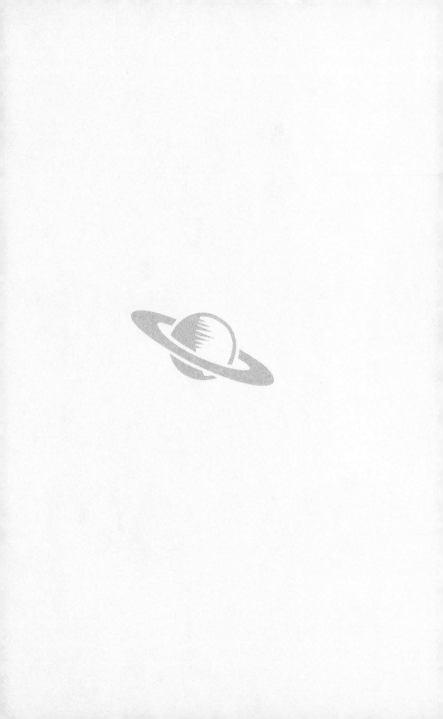

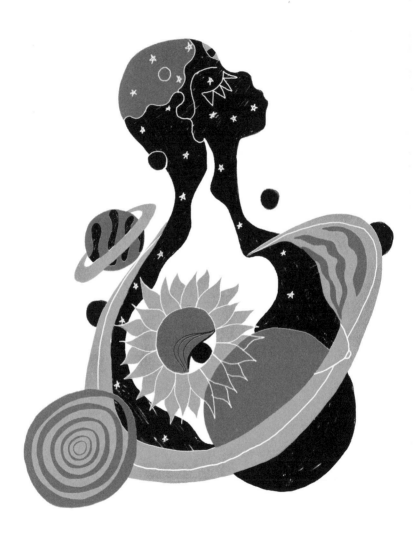

RITUALS

1.39 - "Or by meditating on anything one chooses that is elevating." (Satchidananda, 58)

A unt Tracy, the same auntie who'd later convince me to attend my first yoga class, was also the first one to give me a tarot deck. The deck was her old set of major arcana cards, twenty-two glossy 2.75 × 4.75" cuts of card stock in a silky white drawstring pouch accompanied by an easily digestible reference guide. It was the sort of tarot deck you might get in an airport gift shop and it was her attempt to introduce mysticism to a niece who was more interested in worshipping Rider Strong than in answering life's questions. I recently heard someone say that your first tarot deck should be a hand-me-down, so I guess my story fits with tradition, but it's not like I really gave a shit about tradition. My aunt encouraged me to turn to the deck as a source of stability in my life, but I thought the whole thing was probably complete bullshit.

I mean, I thought the tarot cards were pretty, but I also thought their value was purely visual. I liked displaying my tarot deck in my boarding school dorm room, but only because I thought they made me look cool. But I never actually used the deck for much beyond decoration. I got bored every time I tried to learn how to read them and I limited my practice to intentionally pulling the cards I thought were pretty, like the Lovers. I certainly never explored the meaning of cards that scared me, like Death or the Devil.

For so long, I was unwilling to take spiritual rituals seriously. I used to roll my eyes at anything and everything that could be considered even slightly New Age, including yoga. My Bahá'í beliefs felt more logical than mystical, and I longed for scientific proof that New Age philosophy and spirituality actually "work." I thought spiritual rituals were a waste of time and not to be taken seriously. I attached myself to proof and logic because I feared acceptance of the unknown. I feared what it would mean if I stepped out fully on faith.

God knows when I lost that old tarot deck. I probably gave it to Goodwill somewhere between graduating high school and halfway living out of my car when I first moved to Durham. Anyway, a few years ago, after a Santa Cruz book signing for *Every Body Yoga*, while the bookstore staff folded up chairs and turned down the lights, I wandered the stacks in search of my next book. They'd given me a gift card to say thanks for stopping by, and since I was flying back to North Carolina the following morning, I'd decided to use it before leaving. I started hunting in the spirituality section because my dorky ass obviously wanted yet another book about yoga.

Instead, I stumbled across a very simple red paperback called *How to Read Tarot*, and for some reason I decided to buy it. Then, I found a deck of Marseille tarot cards in the store's sale section. It was a little weird because I couldn't find any other tarot cards in the entire store, and it was the shop's singular copy of *How to Read Tarot*. It felt very meant to be, but I was still pretty skeptical.

I was like, "How do I know this shit is actually real?" How is my perception of what I want out of life not just gonna influence what I read in the cards? And actually, as I learned on the plane ride home the next morning, *How to Read Tarot* directly addressed my quandary in its first few pages. It basically said, "Um, yeah, duh—that's supposed to happen. That's your intuition."

Intuition, aka, the gut punch that made me pick up *How to Read Tarot* in the first place, was something I'd never really valued, even though intuition has guided every step of my life, including and especially this exact moment.

Rituals like tarot and astrology help me use my intuition to understand how order and balance work in the scope of the entire universe. The universe is ratchet and it feels very unpredictable most of the time. Sometimes it appears to work in mysterious ways. But spiritual rituals make things feel a lot less batshit. Or rather, they make the mystery a little fun. They provide structure for the journey of self-acceptance. Rituals create a container for mystical exploration and shine light on the truth that's always emanating from inside of you. Every body is deeply mystical and intuitive. We all have the capacity to engage with our intuition, but capitalism hasn't historically respected it. Instead, capitalism's version of spirituality ignores intuition in favor of materialism.

Ancient rituals help sort through the emotions and baggage that life kicks up. Tarot is like a road map for decoding the path of your life. There are twenty-two cards in tarot's major arcana, and fifty-six cards in the minor. I find both arcana to be very informative, but like the deck that my aunt gave me, some people read only from the major arcana. Each card represents a spiritual phase of human life. Learning to read the cards is an intensely personal journey, and it can provide a lot of context for the moments in your life that can seem otherwise confusing and unmanageable. The meaning of the cards varies depending on how many you've pulled, the order in which they came up, the direction they're facing, and what your intuition has to say about them. The same set of cards read by two different people at the exact same moment will and should have two different meanings, and each meaning is as accurate as the next.

Believing in tarot requires believing in your intuition. If you doubt your intuition, you will always doubt what the cards say. You shuffle the deck, make selections, and decipher their meaning with your intuition. Tarot is not fact-based research, and it'll require wiping that smirk off your face and resisting the urge to second-guess your gut.

I turn to tarot when my eyes can't see, logic fails, and I can't find my next step forward. The cards make that path forward a little brighter.

My mom has been into astrology for literally as long as I can remember. She has journals full of people's readings—anytime a new person comes into her life, she looks up their birthday in one of her many birthday books and reads aloud to them from the pages. She notes their animal totems, their numerology, and their Chinese zodiac signs. She knows everyone's primary elements, whether they're fire, earth, water, or air oriented, and (if the Lord is feeling generous) how those elements work with that of her new friend's partners and children. Me, I gave fewer fucks about astrology and I didn't start really digging into my natal chart until my Saturn started returning. But now, as luck always has it with all of us, I am slowly turning into my mother.

Astrology is a spiritual application of astronomy, the science of celestial objects. Astrology is practical conclusions drawn from the precise locations of astronomical objects. It's a very specific science, but celestial conclusions are not as cut and dry as a horoscope might lead you to think. It's less a prediction of the future than a reading of the present moment.

Horoscopes align your natal chart with each day's unique planetary alignment. Sometimes horoscopes can provide scarily precise intel for deciphering the human experience, but it's usually more fluid and open to subjective interpretation than that. I'm constantly referencing my natal chart and checking my horoscope. I use many different programs, apps, websites, and books to do this.

As I learn more about astrology, new pieces of my natal chart make more sense to me, and I'm able to take comfort in my life's constant fluctuations, as opposed to being pissed that life is impossible to predict and never gonna go according to my plans.

Astrology helps me understand that the divinity that created me is the same divinity that made the galaxy. You and I are made of the same shit that made the moon, stars, planets, and sun. We're imprints of celestial objects walking around on planet Earth, and, like the moon, stars, planets, and sun, our destiny and evolution is charted out in the sky. So it can be helpful to pay attention to what goes on in the solar system, particularly exactly what the sky looked like on the day you were born. Not just the day, month, and year but the exact moment that you emerged. At that moment, the galaxy aligned in an utterly unique way, and you're a reflection of that divine creativity. My girlfriend said it's kinda like we're the performers of stories that have been written by the stars, moon, and planets, and I have to agree. Astrology is a performance of cosmological divinity.

Astrology says that if I pay attention to celestial movements, I can keep in touch with what goes on inside myself. If I accept the ebbs and flows of the solar system, moon cycles, and oceanic patterns, then I can show up more fully to the obstacles of life and understand them as my life's purposes.

I think it's best to just start building your rituals from where you are right now using the tools at your immediate disposal. It's nice to have a special room for doing this shit, but bells and whistles are not required.

I like my sacred space to have stones and sage and plants and flowers and crystals and photos of my loved ones, particularly those who have moved on to the next realm. I've placed crystals and other precious stones all over my home spaces, particularly in my bedroom, yoga room, and office. I regularly wear crystals around my neck or stuff them in my bra. At this exact moment, I'm packing multiple pieces of hematite, jade, and quartz between my titties. I like to wear my crystals in my titties because that way they're closer to my heart.

I keep journals everywhere—in my purse, by the toilet, next to the bed—so I can always write down my emotions as they come up. It helps me contextualize my ocean of emotions as something less than all consuming. I keep Florida water, sage, essential oils, and palo santo handy and maintain a tarot journal for recording my card readings. I keep that same copy of *How to Read Tarot* at the ready so I can reference all the cards that come up. I've got a bunch of different decks now, including goddess, crystal, and affirmation decks. The best days are the ones when I have the time to pull readings from a mix of decks.

I like to blend all my practices and rituals together. I like to lay out all my supplies on or near my yoga mat and move through my practices organically. I think a yoga mat is one of the best places to do a tarot spread because there's actually enough space to spread yourself among the cards. I might start with meditation, transition to journaling, move into a sequence of poses, flow into a tarot card reading before journaling again, and end in meditation. If possible, I keep my phone handy so I can play music and look up anything that comes to mind, as well as reference my horoscope and natal chart (and those of all of my loved ones) at a moment's notice.

Don't think you already know more than what's offered both by the cards and your natal chart. Humble yourself before both the cards and the sky. Think of them as a guide to hearing and understanding what's incomprehensible to your external senses. Use your internal senses to feel what the cards and the stars have to offer.

Value your intuition. It's always giving you the answers to life's questions. One of my great concerns when doing my readings is that I'm misinterpreting things based on my expectations, hopes, dreams, fears, and fantasies. But perception is always colored by these ideas. I'm learning to trust both the process and my gut in equal measure. The answers lie within and not outside me. I have to trust myself enough to hear, see, and feel them. That's how intuition is honed. Honing the intuition brings the present moment into focus.

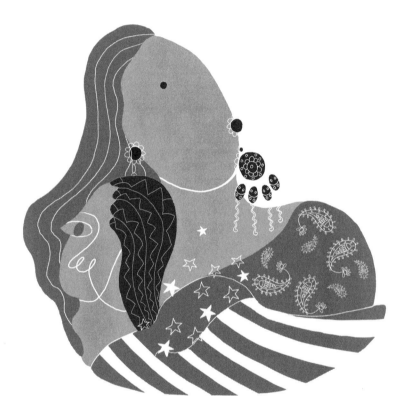

CULTURAL APPROPRIATION IS MORE AMERICAN THAN APPLE PIE

3.6 - "Its practice is to be accomplished in stages."
(Satchidananda, 167)

3.5 - "By the mastery of samyama[5] *comes the light
of knowledge. This means that the truth behind the
object on which we do* samyama *becomes known to
us . . . It's not that anyone creates anything new.
Some truth was hidden. By* samyama, *we understood
what it was. That's the true meaning of discovery."*
(Satchidananda, 167)

---

5 *Samyama* is practice of *dharana* (*concentration*), *dhyana* (*meditation*), and *samadhi* (*contemplation, superconscious state, absorption*) upon one object, usually for the attainment of a particular power (Satchidananda, 227–232).

t's after lunch, about midway through my 200-hour yoga teacher training and I'm laid up in a loose crescent of my fellow trainees. We're on our yoga mats, propped up against back jacks and perched on bolsters, lazily watching a film produced by the founders of Jivamukti yoga. After the screening, our teacher wants us to reflect on one person in the film who'd made a lasting impression on us and find three words to describe that person.

Jivamukti is an American yoga lineage that got a lot of play and popularity in the early aughts because it was considered *the* celebrity yoga practice. This was during an era when yoga became every rich person's national pastime and Jivamukti could be found right at the epicenter of the popularity. Celebrities like Madonna, Sting, Gwyneth Paltrow, and many others devoted themselves to Jivamukti and could be found on talk shows and in magazines proselytizing on behalf of the practice, making certain anyone not residing under a rock would know how Jivamukti had altered their lives for the better.

Most of the film consists of heavily edited interviews with Jivamukti's founders, Sharon Gannon and David Life. Sharon and David were joined in conversation by Willem Dafoe, star of the crime classic *Boondock Saints*, among others. We used to watch *Boondock Saints* on repeat when I was in high school, so I was low-key excited to see Monsieur Dafoe there.

Sharon, David, and Willem were eventually joined by musician Bhagavan Das, and the gang spent most of the film discussing the principles and values of their yoga practices, including scripture, devotion, nonviolence, music, and meditation. They also heavily emphasized the importance of veganism, environmentalism, and social activism. I think some of the film must have been shot in India and I remember hearing Bhagavan Das talk about how amazing it is to *specifically* practice yoga in India because you're immersed in the magic of South Asian cultural heritage.

Equating Eastern spirituality with magic is something White people have been doing for as long as they've been colonizing Asian countries. Countless White colonizers have framed spirituality as a magical offering from Asian people that White people would have no other way of experiencing without appropriating South Asian culture. Since before the nineteenth century, White yoga practitioners can be found making their way to and from India and other Asian countries on spiritual pilgrimages as a way of claiming a deeper connection to their own spirituality.

However, aside from a few random clips of bustling Indian street corners, there were very few actual South Asian people in the video. It was pretty much Whites-only.

The way Sharon, David, Willem, and Bhagavan talked about the practice made me want to barf. It felt as though they'd managed to roll all of the most annoying parts of American yoga culture into one video. Sharon, David, and Bhagavan were all even kitted out in traditional South Asian clothing. As I took in Sharon's sari and bindi, I scrunched up my face in confusion, thinking to myself, "Wait, isn't Sharon Gannon White?"

I quickly remembered that I was absolutely correct and that all the people featured in the video were White. I really can't believe that surprised me because White yoga people seem to *love* wearing South Asian clothing and jewelry, so their behavior was pretty much par for the course. The way Sharon, David, Bhagavan, and Willem were dressed was far from unusual, but it also struck me as remarkably tone-deaf and problematic.

Their behavior reminded me of exactly how White people justify appropriating Black culture. How many times have I heard a White person say some version of "Oh no, it's cool for me to use the word *nigger* when I sing along to Kanye West because my best friend is Black/I fucked a Black girl one time/my childhood maid was Black?" Or "Oh no, it's cool for me to wear kente cloth—my best friend is Black!" This felt like the same conversation in a different outfit. I even made an effort to dismiss my knee-jerk emotional reaction by reminding myself that Sharon and David had undoubtedly spent plenty of time in India, and that at some point during their lives they'd clearly been told it was totally chill for them to dress like the locals. Who was I to tell them how to live their spiritual faith? And what did my desire to criticize them say about how I feel toward myself?

After all, I thought, they represent an untold number of yoga people who appropriate India as their spiritual homeland. They define their yoga practice by the depth of their affinity for South Asian culture. Afterward, they carry the customs of their adoptive homeland back to their OG homeland and spread the word to their patently *non*-Indian friends, thereby strengthening the cycle of normalized cultural appropriation.[6]

I couldn't for the life of me figure out why my teacher was screening a film that might've been produced by the ghost of Rudyard Kipling. It read like a love letter to cultural appropriation and the legacy of British imperialism. It brushed against everything I'd decided to believe about my own yoga practice and I was sure I couldn't possibly be alone. In the age of call-out culture and Twitter punditry, I read the signs of appropriative and imperialistic values as being extremely obvious and I just *knew* my fellow trainees must be coming to the same conclusion.

From my perch in the front row, I craned my neck around the studio and began frantically searching the facial expressions of my classmates. With one eye on the screen, I let my attention wander to the other faces in the room. Surely at least one of them must be having the same level of WTF moment I was having.

---

6 Yes, I'm living the yoga of being a judgmental bitch right now.

I was confused to see that, frankly, no one else seemed to give a shit. Everyone was staring at the screen with facial expressions glazed somewhere on the scale of blank as a pancake to horrifically bored to undeniably comatose. Drool crusted on more than a few lips and at least one person was definitely asleep with her eyes open. Another person was just straight up napping, their light snoring melodically weaving in and around the on-screen dialogue.

I gave up any hope of finding visual camaraderie in my sleeping classmates. Instead, I hungrily searched my teacher's face, trying to discern her intention in screening the film. I reminded myself of the assignment we'd been tasked with and I remembered that we'd already been told the screening would be followed immediately by a guided discussion.

I smiled. That must be why we were watching it! Our teacher must be treating us to this White-man's-burden–ass film to discuss the contradictions it highlighted. I decided our teacher had obviously orchestrated this assignment as a way of teaching us how to sniff out yoga-flavored bullshit. I smiled to myself and decided to turn down my ratchet for the rest of the screening and let my opinions fly during our group discussion.

After the video ended and the lights came up, we each scribbled down the name of someone featured in the film who'd made an impression on us and the three words we'd use to describe them. I gleefully scrawled *Willem Dafoe* on my paper and described him using words like *materialistic*, *self-involved*, and *fake*. I balanced primly atop my roost and awaited discussion with barely contained exuberance.

To my surprise, I was the only one who found the video or any of the people in it to be problematic. While I was only one of many who chose to write about Willem Dafoe, everyone else in attendance described him using words like *relatable*, *centered*, and *authentic*. When I realized that everyone else completely disagreed with my opinion, you coulda caught flies in my mouth.

I didn't realize then what I fully understand now. When my fellow trainees watched that video, nothing about it seemed strange or made them uncomfortable. Because while I found the video to be offensive and appropriative, it actually gave a pretty accurate depiction of how most American yoga practitioners experience yoga culture.

British imperialists treat cultural appropriation as their divine right and the legacy of that mentality is alive and well in American yoga. Cultural appropriation is both an intentional theft of identity and an unavoidable conundrum of the American dream. Cultural *appreciation* means learning and respecting heritage, but *appropriation* always comes down to theft prioritized over reverence. The line between appropriation and appreciation is wafer thin, but acknowledging that line can make the difference between self-acceptance and voluntary participation in Orientalist blackface. Taking on a South Asian "identity" gives American yoga practitioners, especially White people, an opportunity to skirt the shame of their own ancestry by appropriating someone else's. Appropriation morphs the yoga practice into a parody. It becomes yet another way to wear a Mask.

Anyway, when I realized no one else was gonna question the video, I found that my Virgo rising could no longer keep her mouth shut. My hand shot into the air and before my teacher could call on me, I was running off at the mouth about how upsetting and offensive I found the video and how I thought it glorified cultural appropriation and how I was honestly offended that it was part of our YTT curriculum.

Silence. My teacher stared at me without expression. After a moment's pause, she looked me dead in the eye and simply said, "I've never thought of it that way," before abruptly moving on to the next topic.

That bitch shocked me into silence. I was stunned not just by the brevity of her response, but that my reaction seemed to be the first of its kind she'd ever heard. I wanted to argue that it was hard to believe that no other trainee had ever reacted that way in my teacher's near decade of teaching this exact same monthly YTT, but I know a conversational brick wall when I've hit one. Instead of pushing back, I let my voice fall silent. During my rant, I'd felt the emotional bristle of my fellow trainees, and I decided to stop pushing an issue that was clearly making other people feel uncomfortable. After all, what did I expect? I was one of the only Black practitioners in a predominantly White YTT, with an entirely White teaching staff. This reaction should've been far from surprising.

In my silence, I pondered if I was *really* the only trainee who'd ever felt offended by the video. I reasoned that perhaps other trainees had felt the same way but hadn't felt comfortable expressing themselves in such an unwelcoming environment. Maybe they, like I, took cover under the curtain of White acceptance.

In my experience, White people tend to look for ways to categorically deny the effects of White supremacy and cultural appropriation. White people have been led to believe that they don't have a race and are somehow above discussing the subject. In White culture, cultural appropriation and racism are treated like a set of conversational poker chips and weaponry that are exclusively used by people of color when we've got an axe to grind.

In the percussive silence, I was forced to accept that maybe my teachers, especially the White ones, will never feel the way I do about this or any other topic. Whether or not anyone else sees things my way isn't my business. My business begins and ends with my own spiritual journey. I don't need to waste my time trying to convince other people to accept my truth. We're all walking our own journeys in our own time, and the path of another can never be my ministry.

Accepting my own truth is all that matters, and acknowledging the myriad ways appropriation shows up in my own practice isn't easy or pretty. But yoga isn't supposed to feel good or comfortable. It's about understanding what it *means* to be uncomfortable. No one is exempt from the rough edges. The further you go, the uglier it gets. But that can't be a reason to avoid the work.

Yoga transcends any singular—it speaks to a truth that's much bigger than any one cultural identity. It really speaks to the culture of your Self.

The Hindu teachers who brought yoga to America didn't advocate *Hinduism* for the Americans they taught. They advocated *yoga*, freed of religious and cultural context. Yoga naturally leads every practitioner to a deeper exploration of their *own* unique cultural identity. Sprinkling South Asian culture on your yoga practice doesn't make it more legit, it just makes it more appropriative.

Avoiding cultural appropriation means exploring the reasons why we appropriate. Inevitably, it means gazing upon and accepting the colonizer inside of you. This self-exploration is yoga in action.

A few years ago, I was invited to speak on a panel hosted by the National Museum of African American History and Culture. Our discussion topic was cultural appropriation in the worlds of yoga and hip-hop. I was in conversation with an Indian DJ who blends hip-hop and Bhangra. I was extremely nervous because not only was it my first time speaking at a Smithsonian museum, but the other panelist seemed highly critical of American yoga as disseminated by Jessamyn Stanley, a non-Indian Black woman.

My Virgo rising did all she could to prepare, but I had a sneaking suspicion that this panel would end up being atonement by public firing squad for my own cultural appropriation. I felt I was deserving of every inch of judgment that could be thrown by my fellow panelist because I've committed oh so very many culturally appropriative atrocities over the years. I mean, I regularly end my classes by saying the word *namaste*, and I can (sort of) read and write in atrocious Sanskrit. I used to own a yoga mat with a goddamn OM symbol on it. Backstage, I was sweating straight through my Spanx, certain the guillotine was gonna drop at any moment.

But then something weird happened. And that's that absolutely nothing bad happened. The panel ended up being one of my favorite public dialogues—my fellow panelist and I openly interrogated our feelings and theories about cultural appropriation, and I walked out digesting a lot of food for thought. She and I talked about the difference between appropriation and appreciation and how appropriation is usually the result of an absence of respect for cultural heritage. We talked about what it's like to work in industries that are rooted in cultures that are not our own, and it felt really nice for me to connect with someone who has such a specific understanding of my internal conflict and contradictions.

It was really the type of conversation I'd been craving in that Jivamukti screening back in YTT. Truly, it was the kind of conversation that all American yoga schools and media outlets should undertake at every opportunity. Instead of talking about bullshit alignment tips and the best place to get leggings for fall, we should be talking about the hard shit. The shit that can't be accepted without first feeling shame, guilt, embarrassment, and sadness. What it means to appropriate and appreciate a spiritual practice that's based in a culture not native to your own. It doesn't mean beating yourself up about it. It just means being yourself, *all* of yourself, even the parts you don't like.

That reminds me of this time my ex and I were invited to tour Indonesia as guests of the Indonesian US embassy. Everywhere we went, they and I were asked to pose for photos with groups of strangers solely because we're both Black. It became totally normal for locals to approach either us or our Indonesian hosts, gesturing with camera apps and blazing smiles. We'd pose awkwardly, sandwiched shoulder to shoulder with people who were clearly very excited to be standing next to Black people, grinning cheerily and brandishing upturned thumbs and peace signs.

When my ex and I told our hosts that the whole situation made us uncomfortable, they got very defensive. They explained to us that many Indonesians had never seen or met a Black person, and it shouldn't be surprising to us that a few people might want to snap a picture with us. I didn't ask any follow-up questions, but the defensive and slightly embarrassed facial expressions of all our hosts still has me wondering if any of *them* had ever asked to awkwardly pose with a Black person.

And then there was the time I found myself wandering around a very busy Singaporean mall after teaching a class in the same neighborhood. Singapore is hot as hell, and that day I wore my signature hot weather uniform of daisy dukes with a halter top. It was an outfit that would be considered wholly unremarkable back home in North Carolina, but in Singapore, where there are very few Black people, it made me as distinctive as a peacock in a field of reeds. My dark skin and visibly fat body contrasted dramatically with literally every other human being on the premises, and being the only Black person moving through thick throngs of people of color is a sensation I won't soon forget. Plus, openly staring at Black people is (apparently) totally normal in Southeast Asia so literally *everybody* was staring at me. Literally. Staring. Like, kids would stop walking and just stare at me and their parents did nothing to stop them because they, too, had stopped to stare.

I wonder how any of this is different from that Jivamukti video. It reminds me of photos that my White friends from high school post on Facebook of them hugged up on Black kids while studying abroad in Africa. I've always suspected that photos like that are proof of the boundless reach of imperialism and colonialism. But maybe it's proof of more. Maybe there's an imperialist in all of us. Maybe we stare at each other because we don't know what to do when we see someone who doesn't look like us. Maybe sometimes we get appreciation and respect confused with appropriation and colonization because we don't want to look at the patterns. And maybe we weren't always programmed to act this way. But I think we've all been permanently affected by our collective history of White supremacy.

I don't know where all of this leaves us, but I do know that cultural appropriation is not a requirement of practicing American yoga. Yoga will lead you back to your own native culture every time. If you're really reckoning with the light and the dark within yourself, if you're really doing the work of yoking, you will always end up reckoning with the White supremacy that lives inside of you. It's impossible to hide from the truth forever.

There's no easy solution to any of this conflict, and I think that's okay. I don't think you need to find a solution. I think you just have to observe everything that's here, even the parts you don't like. I don't think there's an answer that's not gonna piss off somebody. But I think that's where Acceptance comes in. Your only real option is to just accept the reality of all this. Don't try to change it. Don't try to rationalize it. Don't try to fix it. Just accept it. Then we can all move forward together.

Learn the history. Read the books. Don't pretend to be something you're not. Respect the history of Sanskrit. Respect South Asian culture. Respect what you don't know and respect your elders. Respect that the way you practice yoga has the potential of offending other people. Don't waste time on self-flagellation—learn from your mistakes and move forward.

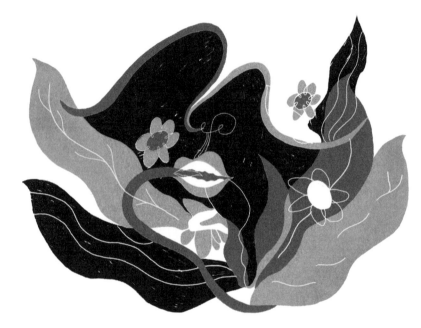

BREATHING

*1.34 - "Or that calm is retained by the controlled
exhalation or retention of the breath."
(Satchidananda, 54)*

Y ou couldn't have paid me to care less about breathing when I first started practicing yoga. I thought it was a waste of my time and I completely disregarded it as a practice. I thought the most important yoga was the yoga of acrobatic over splits and scorpion forearm stands, and I would gladly rush through my breathwork to get to the postural calisthenics that I favored over breathing.

When I did finally start to care, it was only after realizing that applying focus to my breath would strengthen my yoga postures. You really can't practice yoga postures without establishing a strong connection to breathing. Breathing is low-key the only thing that actually matters. When you're in yoga class and shit starts to go south, it's usually because you've stopped breathing. It happens with such a subtle quickness, too, that I usually mistake it for something else. All of a sudden, everything about practicing yoga becomes terrible: the postures are too hard, the teacher's a dick, the room's too hot, my pants are too tight, my mat's too small, the person next to me smells like garbage, the works. But all that really happened was that I forgot to breathe and not breathing made me lose touch with reality.

Breathing is what defines a yoga practice because breathing connects you to the life force that's constantly flowing in and around you. Everything that lives is breathing, and that shared energy is what unites us. You, me, trees, maggots, whales, penguins, Santa Claus—we all breathe. Well, maybe not Santa Claus. But you get the idea.

It doesn't matter if you breathe through tubes, water, or photosynthesis because it's all the same breath. When you intentionally connect to this all-encompassing life force, you're reminded that life is a lot bigger than the jobs you do, the Masks you wear, and the responsibilities you manage.

Find your breath and you're practicing yoga. The posture itself is irrelevant. That means you, me and, everyone we know are always practicing yoga in every posture, whether it's clear to us or not. When you realize yoga isn't just happening when you're on a yoga mat, it becomes clear that the breath is the first thing that should be established in every moment, and not just when you're practicing a sequence of postures. Because, really, every moment in life *is* a yoga posture. Standing up tall when someone's trying to shrink you is a yoga posture. Protecting your loved ones is a yoga posture. Finding the breath in these moments inspires you to action and confirms your faith. Sometimes finding your breath can be the difference between seeing someone else's point of view and punching them in the face.

Finding the breath isn't always simple. Sometimes it can be hard as fuck. I think it's impossible to remind yourself to breathe *too* frequently because there are endless opportunities to forget. Some days it feels like pulling teeth to remember. But to engage with your subtle, spiritual body, you've gotta gain some level of control over your physical body. Postures are one part of how you gain control and pranayama, frequently translated as breathwork, is the other.

Prana is the cosmic energy that's constantly moving through and around all of us. Prana imbalance is the cause of most suffering and it physically manifests as injuries and disease. By controlling prana and how it flows through your body, you can be more aware of and present to all the nerve endings and thoughts within your mental and emotional bodies. When you hold your breath, you retain and restrict the functions of your physical body. Oxygen is the most important component to a functioning human body, and restricting access is literally the quickest way to die. But what happens when you're under stress—what's the first thing you kick to the curb? Breathing. You start holding your breath or refusing to breathe as soon as the panic sets in and the only way to release the sensation is to breathe through it.

Yoga postures filter your breath through your body so that your physical body can find rest for meditation. Breath is the butter that sizzles on your body's cast-iron skillet. Like a cast-iron skillet, your body can cook all kinds of things, but it's gonna need a little fat to get shit poppin'. The breath is the fat.

The body is a vessel that's capable of experiencing and comprehending the deepest mysteries of the universe, but only when it's been seasoned and united with all of its components. When you have control over your physical body, you're able to bear witness to your subtle body. You're able to experience the You beneath your Mask. In this way, pranayama benefits every physical practice—not just traditional yoga postures, but every kind of physical activity. Again, every movement and every life circumstance is yoga in action.

Much of life's anxiety and unhappiness comes from disconnection to your breath. The panic I feel in my anxiety attacks is always cued by not breathing. Reestablishing a connection to my breath is always my first step in dealing with anxiety. I use the same techniques to manage anxiety that I use when I'm struggling with yoga postures. I always return to my breath.

Breath comes first, with all physical and mental action following in its wake. Usually, when a posture or life situation feels difficult or out of reach, it's because my mind is driving and I've thrown my breath in the backseat. The breath helps me understand that the posture isn't out to get me and that, regardless of what it looks like, my body is always getting exactly what it needs.

When a posture or life circumstance challenges or pushes me beyond one of my many predetermined limits, it's never that the posture is out of my reach or that the challenging circumstance shouldn't be happening to me.

It's really that my expectations of what I'm capable of are holding me back from accepting who I am.

If prana is the cosmic energy, then pranayama is the regulation of that energy. You correct your prana imbalances through regulation and retention of your breath. Practicing pranayama, both individually within yourself and collectively with all of creation, means gaining a greater control of the unseen matter that powers you, me, and everything around us.

However, the whole concept of prana is frequently misunderstood in American yoga. I mean, I'm part of the problem. Like most people, I tend to translate the Sanskrit word *pranayama* as breathwork. Breathwork is pranayama's most obvious translation because the most obvious demonstration of pranayama is the way breath passes in and out of your lungs.

But prana consists of much more than air, evidenced by the fact that all living beings share more with each other than just air. Prana is the unspoken connective energetic tissue between all of us. It's everything that fills up the space around you, not just what's visible to your naked eye. Not even air is visible to your naked eye. Prana is the cosmic energy that has fascinated scientists and mathematicians for thousands of years and inspired an untold number of equations and theories.

Prana carries our thoughts and emotions. It's the chariot of our love, hate, fear, sadness, and dreams. You can feel the weight of prana when a room's tension can be cut with a knife, and when the Holy Spirit has entered the building. You can feel it in the heat of a raucous mob and in a natal delivery room. Within the molecules between you and me are our collective emotions, stories, and dreams. You can feel the weight of its presence even if you can't see prana with your eyes. And even though you can't see it with your eyes, if you open your heart, you can feel prana from the inside out. Pranayama is the way all of our energy collides, and while it's one singular collective energy, it's also an infinite number of energies held within an infinite number of physical bodies. Prana holds all of our heartache and all of our joy. It's the very essence of everything. It is *so* much more than the passage of oxygen through lungs.

But America is nothing if not a capitalist experiment, and if there's one thing capitalism doesn't give a fuck about, it's cosmic energy or any of the other fruity shit I was just talking about. In that way, pranayama is rarely, if ever, accurately translated in mainstream American yoga.

In American yoga, capitalism has programmed us to believe only in what can be seen with the naked eye and what can be collectively agreed upon. But everything can't be seen with the naked eye and we're not always gonna agree on everything. Regulating the fluctuations in our cosmic energy is how you and I can start accepting the shit that tears us apart. The breath unites every single piece of all of us. Without control of the breath, you and I will never find unity beyond our perceived differences.

Even though prana is much more complex than oxygen, regulating your breath can help you be aware of the prana constantly flowing in and around you. So even though pranayama is more than just breathwork, breathing is a great way to begin the journey.

It helps if you find the breath before doing anything else. Before making a move, sit your ass down and make a distinct connection with your breath. Even if your yoga teacher didn't say anything about breathing and doesn't encourage you to make a distinct connection with your breath, do it anyway. Go no further without taking a moment to connect with your breath. Depending on the situation, it might be better to breathe entirely through your mouth, entirely through your nose, or a mix between the two.

Some days, finding the breath is gonna feel like trying to find your glasses when they've been sitting on your face the whole time. Especially when you're in the midst of a panic attack, the breath is gonna feel just out of your reach even though it's the first thing you learned how to do. So pretend you're catching your breath for the first time. Find the gumption it took to survive your first moment in this world. You did it once. It only stands to reason you could do it again.

Any posture will work for pranayama. On your back, in a chair, at the office, in bed, or standing up. All postures are the same. The essential work happens along the spinal column so it definitely makes sense to find a position in which the breath can move easily up and down the midline of your body. Common wisdom says to sit upright with the chest open, shoulders relaxed down the back, and the crown of your head shining to the sky. But pranayama should be practiced regardless of your physical posture. If you're practicing at home, don't sweat the specifics of any one posture, just find a position that feels comfortable and sustainable.

There are many methods of practicing pranayama, but I think the best way to begin is by breathing evenly through your nose. Yes, that's all. You probably think you're "above" trying this practice and that it's too simple or easy to be the focus of your attention. I feel you, bitch. I, too, have mistaken pranayama as being too easy to give a shit about. But I promise you're never too advanced to revisit the basics.

Practice simply inhaling and exhaling through your nose. Let your breath rock you like a river rocks a boat. Feel the spots where your inhales are raggedy and rough, and the spaces where your exhales are short and tight. Resist the desire to be judgmental—don't try to *make* your breath do anything. Just be present to what it is, how it feels, how it sounds, and how it tastes. Let yourself linger at the ends and beginnings of your inhales and exhales. The darkness at the ends and beginnings of your inhales and exhales have more to teach than your breath itself. When you return to the basics, you'll realize the naivete in attempting to master something as complex as inhaling and exhaling through your nose. There's no way to master this practice. You'll be a student of pranayama until your final exhalation.

If you want to mix it up, practice breathing for varied numerical counts. Start with inhaling for four counts and exhaling for four counts. Then just multiply or divide from there—inhale for eight counts, exhale for eight counts. Go up to sixteen counts on both sides. Then, when you're tired of that, remix it further—inhale for eight counts, exhale for sixteen counts. Inhale for eight counts, exhale for four counts. If you feel like it, add a few yoga postures. Use the inhales and exhales to move in, out, and around different postures, but let it happen instinctively. This ain't square dance night at the honky-tonk so you don't have to worry about keeping a standard rhythm. Move organically *with* your breath and over time, you'll find that you're moving *through* your breath and that your life force is a manifestation *of* your breath. The breath will become your primary motivator and teacher. It will not only deepen your postural practice and navigate your journey toward meditation, but it will also unearth a stronger connection to your inner and external worlds.

I doubt you'll get bored with inhaling and exhaling for numerical counts. That eight count will become a fascination for you. If you let it, rolling with the breath will feel like swimming through space, with the silence of the solar system pressed against your eardrums. It'll be more interesting than any TV show or book or movie. More interesting than any purchase or music or relationship. In the inhales and exhales, the truth is revealed. And all you have to do is breathe.

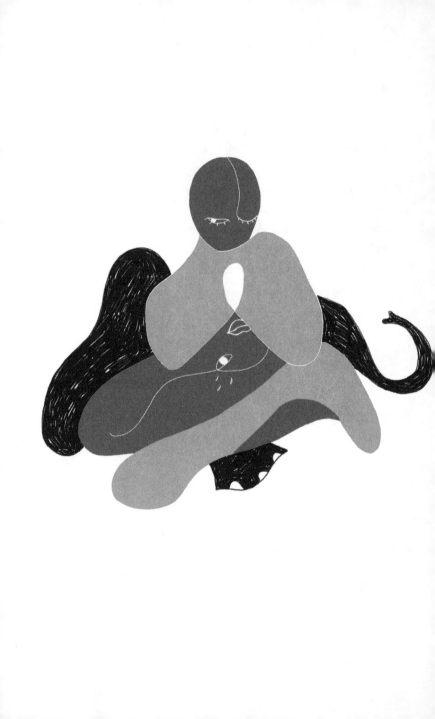

WHITE GUILT

2.5 - "Ignorance is regarding the impermanent as permanent, the impure as pure, the painful as pleasant, and the non-Self as the Self." (Satchidananda, 82)

"A filament gives pure light but appears to be red because of the red glass that surrounds it. Likewise, we are all the same light; but we do not look alike, act alike, or think alike because of the nature of our bodies and mind . . . Through Yogic thinking we can see the entire humanity as our own. We can embrace all without any exceptions . . . We will never criticize a sinner if we realize that we were once in the same boat." (Satchidananda, 104)

"Thus, we take the changing appearances to be the unchanging truth . . . We take the body to be our self; and, speaking in terms of it, we say, 'I am hungry' or 'I am physically challenged'; 'I am black' or 'I am white.' These are all just the conditions and qualities of the body. We touch the truth when we say, 'My body aches,' implying that the body belongs to us and that therefore we are not that . . . Whenever we forget this truth, we are involved in the non-Self, the basic ignorance." (Satchidananda, 82)

"Yoga says instinct is a trace of an old experience that has been repeated many times, and the impressions have sunk down to the bottom of the mental lake . . . When we do something several times, it forms a habit. Continue with that habit for a long time, and it becomes our character. Continue with that character, and eventually, perhaps in another life, it comes up as instinct . . . In the same way, all of our instincts were once experiences. That's why the fear of death exists. We have died hundreds and thousands of times. We know well the pang of death. And so, the moment we get into a body, we love it so much that we are afraid to leave it and go forward because we have a sentimental attachment to it." (Satchidananda, 87)

On the first night of the *Every Body Yoga* book tour, I asked if anyone had one final question, and a very tall Black guy standing at the very back of the house raised his hand. He started out by talking about how much he loves yoga, but how he can never find a sense of calm in yoga studios. He confided that most of the yoga studios he attends are predominantly patronized by White women.

He wondered how a Black man is supposed to find "zen" or "calm" in such an environment. How was he supposed to chill within a predominantly White environment where most of his teachers and fellow students are White women, who society has taught to fear Black men. How was he supposed to find inner calm in a room where he's treated like a threat to his fellow students?

His question definitely caught me off guard. Usually, my Q&As are dominated by questions about how and why a fat person should find ways not to hate themselves, a topic that has always made feel more circus sideshow than yoga teacher. It was the first time anyone had explicitly asked me about the emotional trauma Black people undergo in predominantly White American yoga classes, even though yoga itself is supposed to serve as a balm for trauma.

Perhaps no one had ever broached the topic because quite a few of my students, readers, and followers identify as White or White passing—and White people absolutely hate being reminded of race. When Black people publicly address race, even though we talk about it all the time with each other, it always seems to piss off White people.

As a result, the loudest American yoga voices are much more likely to debate the merits of cotton versus polyblend leggings rather than ever talk about race, especially as it pertains to their own lives. White supremacy lives in all of us and it's a controlling force of American yoga, allowing destination yoga retreats and yoga mat cleansers to dominate mainstream yoga conversations while casting aside racism as an inappropriate and problematic topic.

And yet those same White folks who say they don't like to talk about race are totally chill attending yoga classes taught by me. Now, I'm sure plenty of those White folks would say they "don't see race," which makes no sense to me when every Black person I know seems perfectly capable of seeing race. I think saying you don't see race is just another way of saying you don't want to *talk* about race.

It's cool—I'm not offended that you don't want to talk about race. That's what always happens with taboo topics. Instead of facing them head on, we pretend they don't exist and we get pissed when other people intrude upon our carefully constructed fantasies. In this particular fantasy, slavery never happened and going to yoga classes taught by fatty Black yoga teachers absolves White guilt.

Maybe you're trying to wash away the shame and sins of your ancestors. I don't blame you. White people have repeatedly acted like dicks throughout history and they've attempted to colonize literally every single continent on the planet. Maybe my performance of the magical yoga negro gave clearance for you to ignore this truth even more than you would have otherwise. But that's not actually how it works. Ignoring doesn't make nasty shit go away. It just makes it smell worse when you finally decide to take out the trash.

Well, if we're all admitting things, *I* can admit that I used to seek approval of White folks. Used to? Get real, Jessamyn. YOU STILL DO.

God, that sounds disgusting when I say it out loud, but it's true. I thought there was a seat for me at the White kids table and all I needed was to muster up the confidence to sit down.

The part of me still desperately craving a seat at that table isn't seeking any further inquiry into any of my stank-ass baggage. She wants to be proud of what she's accomplished. She wants to be proud that White people come to her yoga classes. Her heart leaps when events are sold out weeks in advance and she's not bothered when her class attendees are predominantly White, even though her liberal arts education has made her all too aware of how exoticization and fetishization should be included as budget line items for their clear effect on her profit margins.

But it doesn't serve my practice if I only ask questions that feel painless. I've gotta answer the questions that crawl up under my skin and make me want to blend into the wallpaper. I can't decolonize American yoga without decolonizing myself first. I have to decolonize myself as a means of decolonizing the world around me.

In the early days of my yoga practice, I aspired to be the first fat Black person on the cover of *Yoga Journal* magazine, and when the opportunity came knocking, I felt as though all my hard work toward mainstream acceptance (aka White acceptance) had paid off. The day my cover was released, I jumped out of bed and skipped breakfast to immediately drive to the Barnes and Noble periodical section. I scanned all the magazine covers, searching for my face among them. When I came upon the *Yoga Journal* section, I was confused. Because, while I was definitely looking at *Yoga Journal*'s February 2019 issue, I wasn't looking at my face. I was looking at the face and body of Maty Ezraty, the legendary founder of Yoga Works and someone whose likeness epitomizes the idea of a thin, able-bodied, light-skinned person.

In my confusion, I started thumbing through the other issues on the rack. I assumed Barnes and Noble must have made some sort of mistake. Maybe my cover was buried beneath special editions or something. Sure enough, I found a few copies of the edition featuring my photo beneath the Maty Ezraty cover. This didn't dull my confusion. I checked the date on both covers—both were labeled "February 2019." That's when I started to understand that *Yoga Journal* had decided to run two covers and I wasn't the only one being featured.

This was the first that I'd heard about anyone other than me being on the cover, and I scrunched up my brow trying to remember if, in any of the many emails between my management team and *Yoga Journal* in the months prior to pub day, anyone had ever mentioned that anyone else would be on the cover. I didn't want to think the worst.

I didn't want to think that the *Yoga Journal* team, who'd been perfectly cordial during my cover's production, had been potentially racist, deceptive, or exploitative on purpose. I told myself that perhaps they'd decided to show more diversity of practitioners by printing multiple covers. I reminded myself to feel honored that my name was even in the same sentence as Maty Ezraty's, whose teaching practice inspired many of the teachers who influenced my own practice.

I was flustered in the middle of Durham's last remaining Barnes and Noble in the middle of a workday, like I had nothing better to do than stand around feeling foolish. I tried to shake off my sucker punch of emotions by scouring my Gmail inbox to no avail. At no point had anyone ever informed me that anyone else would be on the cover. Why would they hide that information?

In the weeks following the issue's launch, it became clear that I was not the only person with questions. Because my cover had been announced in advance, there were a lot of people who seemed to be as surprised by the double cover as I was. The internet yoga world erupted and battle lines were quickly drawn. On one side, there were people who felt the double cover minimized the impact of *Yoga Journal* finally featuring a fat Black practitioner. They freely used words that generally make White people very uncomfortable, like racism and fatphobia.

On the other side, there were those who seemed annoyed by the outrage. They argued that *Yoga Journal* had every right to run a double cover and that claims of racism and fatphobia were just further proof of snowflake-level hyper social-sensitivity. I wasn't surprised by the battle lines and I felt validated by the perspectives of both camps. I mean, I *knew* that *Yoga Journal*'s actions were proof of both racism *and* fatphobia, but I was also equally aware that most American yoga practitioners choose to ignore the realities of discrimination. The conflict that ensued warmed my inner sociologist's heart. But, instead of standing on a soapbox with my pitchfork held aloft, my inner sociologist grabbed her popcorn and stood at the back of the fray. Aside from occasionally raising my eyebrows or cackling at some of the pettier commentary, I kept to myself and tried not to get involved.

As usual, the universe told my decision to suck a dick. Shortly after World War Yoga commenced, *Yoga Journal*'s editor in chief rang me up. During my cover production, the EIC and I got on like gangbusters. However, I was immediately apprehensive when she hit me up. I knew the sky must be falling at *Yoga Journal* HQ. Not even Richard Spencer enjoys being called racist, and facing a battalion of angry magazine subscribers probably wasn't a fun thing for the EIC to deal with over her morning coffee. Since I grew up around White people who also hate dealing with their White guilt, I knew that their typical reaction to being accused of racism is to brandish the first Black person in proximity, shouting, "How can *I* be racist if I have a Black friend?"

"DO YOU SEE MY BLACK FRIEND?" they say, shaking said friend nearly to the point of death. "She doesn't think I'm racist, so why should you?"

I knew that *Yoga Journal* wanted me to be *their* Black friend. So instead of answering the phone like a grown-up, I freely admit that I hid from *Yoga Journal's* EIC for several days before finally being wrangled into a telephone mea culpa.

I was being passive-aggressive because, frankly, I didn't feel like listening to a White person whine about her White guilt. I knew it wouldn't solve anything or make all that much of a difference. But *Yoga Journal's* EIC was unwilling to accept my passive agression. She made it very clear that *Yoga Journal's* public response to the controversy was on hold until after she'd spoken to me. Grumbling and complaining, I crawled out of my shell and finally submitted to a phone call.

The EIC immediately confirmed that *Yoga Journal* hadn't informed me of the double cover in advance and she apologized profusely for what she deemed an inexcusable lapse in judgment. I suppressed a yawn, and I felt my mother slap me on the thigh. *You don't need to be rude*, she hissed at me. I grumbled an apology under my breath and straightened up in my seat.

The EIC went on, explaining how *Yoga Journal* had decided to show a wider expanse of practitioner diversity by featuring more than one teacher on the cover. She lamented the controversy and said she was very disappointed about how all of the internet noise had distracted attention from my success of being on the cover. She said she'd hoped my feature would start some of the necessary conversations that are rarely featured in the yoga world. She wanted *Yoga Journal* to be the catalyst for those necessary conversations, and she felt that the cover controversy distracted from the work that needed to be done.

I tried to listen patiently, keeping my responses minimal and relatively boilerplate. I told her that while I wasn't expecting the double cover, I wasn't shocked, either. This wasn't the first time that my successes have been minimized by predominantly White institutions. High school, undergrad, and graduate school already stole that virginity. I didn't press her as to why they didn't tell me about the double cover in advance because I'd already realized why they hadn't told me. I knew they'd tried to avoid a difficult conversation.

Yeah, that's right. The magazine that wanted to be a catalyst for difficult conversations had avoided having a difficult conversation with its own token. I found it deeply ironic that the EIC felt the controversy distracted from important conversations in the yoga world because I felt exactly the opposite. I felt *Yoga Journal* had catalyzed the EXACT conversation about racism and fatphobia so *obviously* needed by the American yoga world.

In the days following the cover debacle, I was forced to question why I'd ever been so desperate for *Yoga Journal*'s approval. *Yoga Journal* is a historically White institution. Without consciously thinking about it, I'd hinged my entire identity on the approval of White voices. Why did I need the approval of historically White institutions? Did I think the proximity to Whiteness would prove something about me? Would it make my yoga practice more valid or important or worthwhile?

What does it mean for the grandchild of African slaves to find solace in an American yoga practice that's firmly rooted in the soil of White supremacy? My ancestors were beaten and murdered for indigenous spiritual practices that frightened their enslavers. They found refuge in the versions of Christianity that least offended those that imprisoned them. Just like them, I've found a connection to my spiritual identity via the White man's approved version of spirituality.

At what point should I consider myself a minstrel show? Is it only because I don't wear blackface that I'm able to ignore the comparison? Is the line drawn at inspiring others? Does inspiration negate a minstrel show? At what point do I accept the spectacle that I've allowed others to expect from me? Yoga has led me to question everything. Pandering to the amusement of White folks is the same respectability politics in new clothing.

Why was I so cool with being *Yoga Journal*'s token, anyway? Why did it take so long for me to be pushed to the edge of self-disgust? Maybe it doesn't matter how long it took. But wanting to see myself on the cover was *very* telling of my obsession with being seen and acknowledged by other people. What does that say about how I see myself?

I thought that being on the cover would mean that I'd attained a prize of being close to Whiteness. That it would heal the part of me that has never felt "Black" enough. The part that hid her Jewel and No Doubt albums. The part that was called an Oreo. But it didn't. It only magnified the shame of my assimilation and the White supremacy that lives inside of me.

Like most American yoga teacher trainings, my yoga teacher training center had a predominantly White teaching staff and studentship. I was one of two Black people in my YTT and the only visibly fat person. I think there's a direct correlation between the Whiteness of YTTs and the racism of American yoga. Predominantly White yoga teaching environments breed a species of groupthink that's marbled with White supremacist values. Yoga people of color are less likely to feel supported by predominantly White yoga communities and are less likely to sign up for training programs, which limits the overall diversity of American yoga teachers. Multiplying this equation by every major international city has resulted in a global yoga teaching community with a White supremacist backbone.

White yoga people generally don't consider themselves racist because they prefer to hide behind coconut water etiquette. Coconut water etiquette is repeating shit like *namaste* so loudly and resolutely that no one ever forces you to acknowledge the legacy of racism and genocide fully embedded in American yoga's foundation. But in my experience, there's no amount of coconut water etiquette that can mask racism's foul-ass odor.

Frequently, these same White yoga people claim they want their classes and studios to be more diverse and not so White. But they fail to see how coconut water etiquette undermines this goal. It's *because* they refuse to acknowledge their White guilt that their classes and studios are already not diverse. They refuse to gaze upon their ancestral shame.

I feel that shit. I don't like looking at my inner racist, either. But sooner or later, it's gotta be time to clean house. Mucking out your house isn't fun, but that's okay—not everything in life is about having fun. Sometimes life is cleaning up nasty shit. And racism is some nasty shit.

That guy at my book signing had a point. It's hard to feel chill when no one wants to acknowledge the big-ass racist elephant in the room.

Sometimes White yoga people will shrug off discussions of racism by insisting we focus our self-exploration upon the *whole* self instead of getting hung up on our physical self. And in the same breath, these same practitioners obsess over postural practice, aka the yoga of physical body mutilation.

And that's why I'm done talking to White yoga people about race. They don't want to hear about it and they get mad if you bring it up. They don't think it needs to be discussed and they don't think it has anything to do with their lives or practices. It's not my job to educate anyone about how racism affects all of us, all the time, because it just *does*. It simply does. Whether you like it or not.

Everything in our world starts and ends with race. Even the things that seem unrelated are inevitably somehow tied to race and power. Until we accept that racism lives at the core of our global society, we've got no hope of unity. And I know that, historically and etymologically speaking, racism is White people's game and it's White people's problem to solve. But I would argue that White supremacy exists as a cultural and spiritual genocide. It's filtered into each of us to the point where now, we're all racist. Racism only begets more racism and it's a problem we have to solve together. All of us. Literally everyone. And I see you, Black person who believes we can't be racist. But let's you and me agree to disagree.

There's a part of me that doesn't want to say we're all racist because I know White people will use any excuse to avoid acknowledging the full breadth of their ancestral shame. They'll make it seem like they're no more liable than anyone else. But just because we're all racist doesn't mean that White people don't need to do the heavy lifting of accepting its generational effects. Pay attention to what's said (and unsaid) by your family members, colleagues, and yourself. Hear the things you don't say in mixed company but absolutely think in your head. Think of the things your grandparents said around the dinner table. Feeling embarrassed and ashamed is not enough. Those emotions are not the final answer.

We're not all having the same experience and that's okay. We've gotta stop expecting other people to understand where we're coming from because they just never will. If *you* can't accept where you're coming from, how the hell can anyone else? We're strangers even to our closest friends. What makes us the same is that we're *all* having our own unique experience of self-exploration and acceptance. That's the thread that'll always stitch us together.

You can't accept yourself without accepting that there are collisions at the intersections of your identity. Racism is one such collision. It's not fun to look at and it sucks to accept that you're part and parcel of a system that disenfranchises all of us. Self-flagellation is unnecessary: It doesn't help anyone if you beat yourself like a dead horse. But you can't pretend that the Truth doesn't exist.

I don't think there's a way to fix American Yoga's racism problem. I think there's only acceptance of what is. Maybe once we accept what is, we can find a way to move forward together.

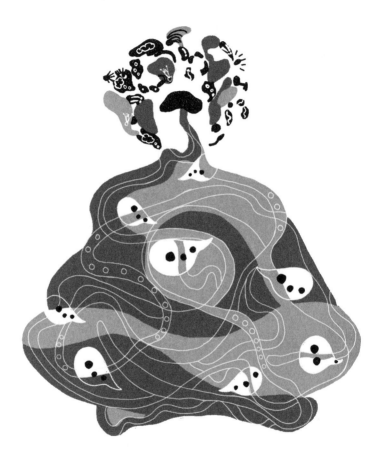

MEDITATION

1.41 - "Just as the naturally pure crystal assumes shapes and colors of objects placed near it, so the yogi's mind, with its totally weakened modifications, becomes clear and balanced and attains the state devoid of differentiation between knower, knowable, and knowledge. This culmination of meditation is samadhi." (Satchidananda, 60)

2.10 - "In subtle form, these obstacles can be destroyed by resolving them back into their primal cause [the ego]." (Satchidananda, 88)

2.11 - "In the active state, they can be destroyed by meditation." (Satchidananda, 88)

1.27 - "The word expressive of Isvara[7] is the mystic sound of OM [OM is God's name as well as form]." (Satchidananda, 40)

1.28 - "To repeat it with reflection upon its meaning is an aid." (Satchidananda, 44)

---

7 *Isvara* is the supreme cosmic soul; God (Satchidananda, 228).

thought I was bad at meditation. I'd resist even trying because I convinced myself that my mind was too busy to find stillness. I thought meditation was only for people who trade in giant jugs of water at health food stores. I've never been a giant-water-jug trader, so I supposed that meditation was not for me.

Truth be told, I hoped I was incapable of it. I wanted an excuse to let myself off the hook. Every time I'd sit down to meditate, I spent most of my time reminding myself not to open my eyes, mentally counting down the seconds until I could stop feigning stillness.

I knew meditation was a huge part of yoga, but I thought there must be a loophole to get me out of doing it. Kinda like trying to determine if I had enough prereqs to get out of a required class.

I didn't take the practice of meditation seriously. And it really is a practice, not a perfect. At its core, meditation is a practice of contemplation. You can practice it all the time. Every moment of life is a meditation. When you're meditating, you can't tell what's up or what's down, and time becomes irrelevant because you're so consumed by the present moment. And there's no way to be bad at it. Or good at it, for that matter.

But I didn't understand that. I thought meditation was just another part of my life that I needed to pretend. Meditation became a box to check off, an assignment to finish on time. Another Mask to don. I gave my meditation practice about the same amount of attention that I gave book reports in elementary school. I knew the practice was good for me because my teachers said so, but I didn't understand how to actually *live* it. I fell in and out of my practice because I believed meditation was beyond my ability.

It's probably fair to say that I found my meditation practice when I stopped looking for it. I'd been consistently practicing different meditation techniques and there were a few guided meditations that became like prayer for me. But I found myself feeling dependent on the voices of my teachers to essentially hypnotize me into something akin to stillness.

One day I decided not to hit Play on my favorite YouTube meditation before closing my eyes. I didn't decide upon a specific breathing technique or tool. I just plopped my ass down, closed my eyes, and sat there. My thoughts crashed in and around me like waves, body-slamming my subconscious from every direction.

But I didn't try to get rid of them. I didn't try to categorize things. I just let all my thoughts be there. I just let all of *me* be there. And not even my most selfish, secretive, schadenfreude-lusting identity was to be turned away.

A mind that moves quickly is meditation's *only* prerequisite, and authentic stillness only comes when you stop trying to pretend it. In my experience, half the difficulty of meditating is created by *pretending* to meditate. I didn't know that I needed to stop being so desperate for the fantasy of calm and just allow the chaotic thoughts to crash in.

Because stillness *isn't*, really. It's the space *between* the trembles. The spot where everything comes together. It's not a final destination. It's the ends of the inhales and the ends of the exhales. It's the moment when you've said I can't take this anymore. It's the space where everything collides. Stillness is oft lost because you're looking for it where it can't be found. You look for it in games of make-believe. You pretend stillness and perform calm, and they become your sock and buskin. All that pretending gets in the way of experiencing the stillness that's always around you. Only when you stop judging yourself and let all your thoughts flood in will the stillness come. The stillness lives between the cracks in your chaos.

When you were a baby, before you knew words, you knew how to meditate. Babies meditate all day long. It's not like they have a lot of options. Where they gon' go? What else are they gonna do, brush up on their French and check their stock options? Nah, bruh. Silent self-reflection and boundless observation of the outside world is an infant's wheelhouse. So you spend the whole first chunk of your life in constant meditation, but you get distracted by a need to communicate with other people. Finding the right word to express your thoughts becomes more important than anything else. And that's where the trouble starts. You get so caught up trying to listen and communicate with others that you forget to listen to yourself. But babies are just little humans, and little humans grow into big humans who still hold the same arsenal of techniques. You and I already know how to do this work. It's really just a matter of remembering.

You and I are still crying infants, and settling into meditation is kind of like quieting the screaming infant that's still inside of you. Except now you're crying about shit that's much scarier than anything you cried about when you were a baby. More often than not, we talk incessantly so we can ignore our internal dissonance. But it's only when you stop talking that you can hear and accept the cacophonous thunder rumbling inside of you.

Meditation isn't something that's only for certain people or certain situations. Meditation is literally the chemical reaction between pranayama and poses. It can and should be utilized by anyone who breathes. No one has a monopoly on meditation. Yes, the concept of meditation is way trendier now than it's probably ever been before. But I think that's a good thing. I think meditation should be the most normalized and basic practice on Earth. Just think about what it means. It really just means extended thought, reflection, contemplation. What's the opposite of meditation? Overlooking, disregarding, ignoring. You and I live in a world where overlooking is glorified. Disregard is a virtue. Ignorance is everyone's favorite defense mechanism. Meditation requires the exact opposite. It means *not* looking away. It means not ignoring. It means nothing can be overlooked. Imagine a world where you haven't been conditioned to disregard. Where you're not desensitized to everything on the table. In this world, you and I don't ignore our differences. You don't disregard pain and suffering.

Meditation looks more peaceful than it feels. Our thoughts aren't meant to be peaceful. They're aggressive, unpredictable, and all-consuming. The point isn't to manufacture quiet. Life is meant for living, and living is suffering and chaos. You're supposed to have thoughts, and they're chaotic by nature. The point is to *accept* your chaos. When you accept your chaos, it gets a lot easier to put shit in order. Marie Kondo always says you've gotta make a big pile of mess before you can organize your house. You've gotta see and accept your chaos in order to get it in check.

Everything you do is preparation for meditation, and meditation is preparation for everything you do. In sickness and in health. In war and at peace. Every breath, every posture, every drop of sweat—everything your physical body does is preparing itself for meditation.

You don't have to practice a bunch of postures to meditate. It really only takes one. No matter how your body looks or moves, there's a meditative posture that'll work for you. A lot of people choose to sit, but you could lie down or stand up.

Here's how I taught myself to practice meditation. Initially, I'd just practice sitting quietly for a few minutes. For me, that was plenty of work. I enjoy meditating with my eyes closed, but that might not feel natural to you. With my eyes closed, I focus on inhaling and exhaling through my nose. I like to set a timer because it helps silence the part of my mind that's obsessed with how long I've been sitting, how long until it's over, and whether or not I've actually got time for this shit. That's one of my go-to inner monologues when I practice meditation—I try to convince myself that I don't really have time to do it and I need to stop as soon as I can.

Gradually, I started practicing five- to ten-minute guided meditations, and eventually transitioned to fifteen- to twenty-five-minute guided meditations. I found a few teachers online who I still love, and I carry their teachings around inside of me. But it didn't take long before I started to feel a bit hemmed in by guided meditations and instead I started setting my phone timer for five- to fifteen-minute unguided meditations. Over time, five to fifteen minutes has grown into forty-five minutes and beyond.

It's hard to describe what meditation feels like, so I'm hesitant to even try. All the words that come to mind sound like utter bullshit when I type them out. One of my favorite teachers has even explicitly said not to try to tell anyone about it because, he says, the feeling is wordless and nameless. I guess more than anything I feel unbothered. I feel like I'm just being.

I don't really think time duration matters all that much. When I'm meditating, whether it's for a few breaths or longer, I'm not all that aware that I'm even meditating. Time starts to feel irrelevant. It doesn't feel like time stands still. It's more like time doesn't matter at all. As though there's an infinite amount of it. As though I can sit for an infinite amount of time because I am able to (finally) just Be.

So much of my life is ruled by time—and not having enough of it. So to *not* notice time feels very remarkable to me.

It usually takes me at least fifteen to twenty-five minutes to fully arrive in meditation. As my breath whooshes in and out, it steadies the fidgets of my physical, emotional, and mental bodies and weaves them into harmony.

I've always heard the mental experience of meditation described as being akin to your thoughts passing over the sky of your mind in the same way clouds cut across a blue sky. You don't try to hold on to the wisps and swirls and puffs because they're just condensation in disguise. Instead, like the clouds crossing the sky, you just acknowledge that your thoughts are there and let them pass by.

The blue sky is a pretty apt description, but for me, meditation feels like swimming in water that's very dark and very deep. At first, it feels like I'm just skimming across the surface of the water. As I establish my breath, it's like my strokes are clipping the meniscus. But the deeper I swim, the more my breath transitions from earthly to aquatic. As I swim deeper within myself, my gills open up and the depth of the water presses against my consciousness. The water is so deep and dark that I don't know if I'll ever reach the bottom. It's scary, but it's also comforting and a little exciting. Like coming home after being away for a very long time.

It doesn't really matter how long you sit in meditation. The amount of time you need fluctuates every day. Don't get hung up on the details. Let it all be fluid and amorphous. The more aware you are of time duration, the less present you're able to be in this moment. As long as you're aware of how long you've been meditating, you're not really engaged in the practice.

I used to think meditation was more like a lobotomy than anything else. But it's nothing like a lobotomy. It's also not really something you can teach other people to do. Regardless of how much guidance you receive from other people or the tips and tricks they offer, you'll always end up training yourself to practice meditation. Whether you're alone on your yoga mat, or you've paid money to sit in front of a teacher. You cannot pay for introspection. Teachers can *guide* your meditation, but they're really just giving you the clearance to teach yourself. They're like a parent holding a child's hand while crossing the street. The kid won't always need that hand but it's helpful for the time being.

Meditation is a state of being—both a noun and a verb. Like yoga, it's a journey and a destination. It's not about scholastic achievement. You may not be able to purchase the ability to meditate, but every moment of life is an opportunity for practice. Especially the moments that don't seem suited to the task. The ideal time for meditation is when you're under duress and the sky is falling. When your heat is rising, the best thing you can do is sink into meditation. Meditation is the ideal response to every conflict and every moment of doubt.

Meditation doesn't mean that your brain is supposed to be silent. If your brain is silent, that means you're dead. Meditation means accepting that your brain is always moving. You have greater control over your well-being because you can observe your thoughts without them taking over your existence. Stillness bookends your inhales and exhales. Chaos is why you're here and meditation allows for acceptance.

Every time I sit down to meditate, my thoughts, fears, and dreams perch on the telephone lines of my mind. As I breathe, they squawk at me. Sometimes I get so annoyed by their squawking that I can't help but angrily stare at them. They stare back at me. One of them shits on my head. But I don't try to shoo them away. I let them exist, exactly as they are.

In those moments there's no choice but to feel it all. I can't hide from my truth, and tears are only my first step. I can no longer stem my ocean. And as the ocean of me erodes the sandcastles of my identity, the Voice inside reminds me to breathe. Just Breathe. Nothing more, nothing less. If I breathe, I can survive.

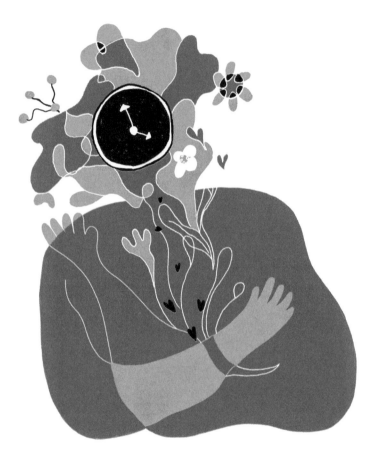

IT'S A FULL-TIME JOB LOVING YOURSELF

"Every time we cover the dirt, it comes back.
When we realize this, we develop an indifference
toward the body; not that we neglect it, but we no
longer adore it. The time we once spent on our bodies
can be used for other purposes like japa,[8] meditation,
or reading spiritual books." (Satchidananda, 134)

"On the level of form, you are not the same person
now as you were last week. Even a minute ago you
were different. Every minute the body is changing:
some part is dying, and some part is being born."
(Satchidananda, 111)

"A happy or unhappy life is your own creation . . .
You are your own best friend as well as your
worst enemy." (Satchidananda, 93)

2.1 - "Accepting pain as help for purification, study of
spiritual books, and surrender to the Supreme Being
constitute Yoga in practice." (Satchidananda, 75)

---

8 *Japa* is repetition of a mantra (Satchidananda, 228).

My first colonic was a belated twenty-ninth birthday gift to myself. I gained weight while writing *Every Body Yoga*, and my mother recommended that I combat this development by seeing a colon hydrotherapist in Mooresville.

Colon hydrotherapy, otherwise known as anally flushing your intestines with jets of lukewarm water, relieves bloating and gas that's caused by consuming digestively disruptive food. All the late nights and early mornings I spent hunched over my keyboard meant I was inhaling french fries and enriched bread like they were going out of style. In response, my body started acting like Violet Beauregarde's in *Charlie and the Chocolate Factory*. And even though my skin didn't turn blue, my body definitely inflated like a ripened berry.

As much as I hate the feeling of discomfort that comes from eating shit my body rejects, I kind of enjoyed my weight gain. I like being soft. I think my body is sexy and I think it's sexy *because* it's fat. Plus, I really love eating, especially eating out in restaurants. My family could rarely afford to eat out when I was a kid, and I still like to celebrate my inner eight-year-old by taking her out for a feast now and again.

Trouble is, I was gaining weight and I wasn't the only one who noticed. My social media followers had only ever seen me as the "slim fat" yoga bitch I presented to the world, and my slide into the world of "full fat" was noticeable. And, as much as I'm ashamed to admit it, it became a big deal to me, too. Even though I felt at home in my fuller figure, I found myself backsliding into the same cycles of anti-fat fuckery that put my ass on the path of self-acceptance in the first place.

By the time I got into yoga, I'd eaten my fill of diet culture's bullshit. I was a textbook yoyo dieter all through my undergrad years, but by the time I got into yoga, I'd pretty much given up on the endless rat race of weight loss. I was reading the works of Lesley Kinzel, Marianne Kirby, and Virgie Tovar, and I started trying to define body acceptance for myself.

Around the same time, I was accidentally living a healthy lifestyle. Every day I rode my bike up and down the hills between me and my grad school classes. I sort of paid attention to my diet and by that I mean I ate a lot of salads and tried to avoid fast food.

Within the first four years of my yoga practice, I gradually lost at least fifty pounds. My memory is left to guesstimations because I broke up with scales around the same time and it's been damn near a decade since I've weighed myself without a doctor present. My weight loss had everything to do with being too cash-strapped to afford groceries for more than a single meal each day. Post-collegiate abject poverty is one hell of a diet plan.

During that time, I spent nearly every night working in one of Durham's busiest restaurants. At work, I layered several pairs of ripped Spanx to minimize thigh chafing as I hurtled through the restaurant's crowded aisles. However, the effect of wearing multiple pairs of Spanx in a sweaty work environment proved to be the equivalent of wearing Khloe Kardashian's tightest waist trainer for hours at a time. All of a sudden, my waist was snatched, my chin was violently sharp, and my collarbone visibly jutted out of my chest.

For the first time since the early days of my adolescence, my weight dipped below two hundred pounds. I spent my mornings sweating out hours of yoga postures before putting on my spandex corset and essentially running a 5K in a restaurant that, depending on the drunkenness of its patrons, regularly fluctuated in temperature from eighty to one hundred degrees Fahrenheit. I developed the breasts of a seventies porn star and I bought bras in sizes even smaller than what I'd worn as a teenager.

Since quitting my restaurant job to focus on teaching yoga, the weight I lost in the early days of my practice has gradually crept back and multiplied. As I write you, I'm the fattest I've ever been in my life. But since I've *always* identified as Fat, even when I was a kid, the weight gain hasn't felt like a big deal to me. If anything, it's felt like a return to form, like shedding this weird thin skin I grew in my twenties and returning to who I was before I learned how to hate myself. Being thinner never felt familiar to me. It always felt abnormal, like the greatest Mask of all. Honestly, until other people started telling me I looked fatter, I hadn't even noticed that I *was* thinner. In my thinnest years, I distinctly recall thinking

I looked then exactly as I do right now. But projecting my latent self-hatred onto other people? That's familiar. That's a tune I've been singing for a very long time.

It turns out that no matter how much body positivity I ingest, I'm nothing but a fatphobic slut-shamer just like the rest of you. Why wouldn't I be? Body negativity is basically an American value at this point. To love your body is to stand in direct opposition to capitalism. Plus, it's really not that hard to love your curves when your body shape is cosigned by the fantasies of White cis masculinity. A love of my curves doesn't make me any less plagued by fatphobia and self-hate. Accepting the curves that White supremacy cosigns does not equate to body liberation. It just means I've got more boxes that need to be deconstructed.

My body positivity has only ever extended as far as White supremacy will let it. It's proof that capitalism has figured out how to monetize a commodified version of my Truth. Beneath adoration of my fat ass and thick thighs lies unresolved resentment toward the parts of my body that I haven't been granted permission to accept. When the demons come, I still find myself wrestling with my physical body.

It's not brave to live in your own skin, especially not when your body is the new average. And by this point, life as an unapologetic US 18 should be beyond the norm.

What's hidden at the root of my professional success is an insidious belief that if a fat Black person can find a way to love themselves, then "regular people"[9] *must* be capable of self-love. I think this is supposed to make me feel fulfilled and satisfied. I think I'm expected to find my life's purpose in the idea that anyone would care enough about my yoga practice to catch it on film. Even if they're only filming it with the same supremacist curiosity that stirs the audience at SeaWorld.

The language of Fat is really what scares people. Everyone, we Fats included, has been trained to think *Fat* is a dirty word. When I call myself Fat in a room full of non-Fats, it's like firing a shotgun. Once the smoky silence clears, non-Fats always leap to correct my language. "You're not fat, you're beautiful!" is their endless refrain. I shrug my shoulders, amused by the obvious awkwardness. I simply said I was fat. I never said I wasn't beautiful, too.

Fat Blackness is only allowed in the mainstream when it's controlled by Whiteness. But what happens when my yoga stops making thin White people feel good about themselves? What happens when their mammy complexes are thrust into the spotlight? What happens when my body positivity stops being about them and (finally) starts being about me? How long before they realize I'm the fat nigger they've been taught to fear?

---

9 Read: thin White people.

What happens when my body positivity disgusts them? What happens when my yoga disgusts them?

Common wisdom says we Fats should limit ourselves. It discourages us from trying new things, stepping out of boxes, or even accepting Fat identity as part of our Truth. There's a cultural disease that wants us to believe our bodies do not belong to us and the White man's body positivity ain't enough to bridge the divide. There's no *solving* Fat identity: only acceptance.

But what *I* underestimated about body acceptance is that it's never as simple as accepting what your body *looks* like. Accepting your body means accepting all the things it's done—*and* all the things that have been done *to* it.

After #MeToo started trending, you couldn't get on social media without reliving somebody else's trauma. And I was surprised to find that when I came upon unsolicited survivor stories, I wasn't happy to see them. I couldn't believe how angry they made me. It turned out my progressive Black feminism had strings attached. I got mad when other people were brave enough to tell their stories because their memories triggered my own.

It's March 2012 and I'm riding Megabus home from New York City. I took Megabus a lot in those days.

It was one of those all-night rides where you board in Midtown Manhattan and travel through the night to North Carolina, stopping once in DC and then once again in Roanoke.

I don't remember when he sat down next to me. It must have been after we stopped in Roanoke. I don't remember much about him other than he smelled like the dregs of the Four Loko can he was concealing in his coat pocket and surreptitiously snatching sips from in the shadows. He made me feel a little uncomfortable but he also seemed relatively harmless so we struck up a conversation that I tried to end by pretending to fall asleep. When he saw that I was nodding off, he leaned his head against my shoulder and asked if it would be okay for him to "sleep lean" on me. "Sleep lean" furniture is a frequent unspoken trade of fat people, so it felt harmless to oblige him. Maybe he would leave me alone if he could find a comfortable sleeping position.

He snuggled up closer as we bumped like Yahtzee dice through the Virginia countryside. That's when I started to tense up. This didn't feel right. All of a sudden, his hot-ass breath was right next to my ear and his hand had somehow fallen atop my torso.

"Is it okay if I rest my hand here," he mumbled. Full stop. No question mark.

Surely my perception was being scratched on a record. How could a complete stranger feel justified in touching me so intimately? I mentally fumbled through a slate of responses, but my good little Bahá'í girl travel phrasebook was ill-equipped for this kind of diplomacy.

I immediately blamed myself. I reasoned that our earlier banter must have given the impression that I would find his touch welcome. It must have been my fault, I thought. I must have been too nice. I feared the awkwardness that would descend by verbally rebuffing his advances so I reasoned that Silence was a perfectly legitimate response. I continued to feign sleep and prayed that Silence would convey my wishes.

Please don't touch me, I Silenced at him.

I don't like this, I Silenced at him.

I don't know you, I Silenced at him.

Please don't touch me.

Instead of heeding my Silence, I felt the stranger's hand crawl up my sweater and before I could process my next move, his hand was roughly squeezing my bare breast.

Breathing became superfluous. How could this possibly be okay, I Silenced. How could I get it to Stop. What had I done to invite This.

As usual, my self-hate was ruthless.

She said, "You dummy. Your silence is your invitation."

Shamed in the heat of her gaze, I wondered what would happen if I cried out. But what if he gets *more* violent? I didn't know what to do. I felt like a deer in headlights. I reasoned to myself that if I pretended to be asleep, it'd all be over much quicker.

I don't know how long it went on. As I felt him dozing next to me, I put my body on autopilot and my mind wandered. I waited for his grip to slacken and started to shimmy out of his grasp, but his grip tightened as soon as I moved. He spent the rest of the trip trying to snuggle against me and *I* spent the rest of the trip struggling against him, trying to turn my body at any angle that might make touch less accessible. But every time I flinched or shifted, he'd tighten his grip.

By the time we pulled into the Raleigh bus depot, all I wanted was to go home and never ride Megabus ever again. I was already desperately trying to file the incident in the back of my mind. It wasn't the first time something like this had happened to me, and I had every intention of putting it in the same mental cardboard box on the same shelf in the very back of my mind where I hide everything that scares me.

The Stranger skulked around me while I collected my luggage, asking about my plans now that we were back home.

I told him my boyfriend was collecting me and I'd better wait for him outside rather than wait inside the bus depot. Southern predators rarely hear the word "girlfriend" the same way they hear the word "boyfriend," so I usually claim to have a boyfriend when I don't feel safe. This was in the days before Uber, so I hid behind the depot until I saw my girlfriend's car approaching. I considered catching one of the cabs that idled in the taxi lane instead, but I knew I didn't have enough money to pay for a ride. When I was finally buckled in the passenger seat of my girlfriend's car and we were pulling away from the depot, I burst into tears but couldn't wrap my mind around how to tell her why. I doubt I ever did.

A few years later, during *Every Body Yoga*'s press tour, I traveled to the Tribeca Film Festival to attend a screening of a mini-documentary about my yoga journey. I arrived at my hotel within an hour of the screening, only to be told that my room was not yet prepared. I ended up getting dressed for the soiree in the hotel's public restroom. While the hotel restaurant's breakfast crowd freshened up, I steamed my gown, wrangled my FUPA into Spanx, and tried not to block the paper towel dispenser while applying my eyeliner.

After the screening, as I finally made my way up to my hotel room, I remember saying hello to one of the hotel's doormen I'd met during a previous stay. He was jovial and playfully flirtatious. While unpacking, I received a call from the front desk: apparently, there was a package waiting for me. A few minutes later, someone knocked—it was the jovial and playfully flirtatious doorman.

He handed me the package and immediately started chatting me up. I did my best to be polite, but I was late for a date with Postmates and Netflix and couldn't care less about whatever the fuck he was talking about. I escalated from subtle verbal cues to shutting the door in his face. But the jovial and flirtatious doorman wouldn't budge. Eventually, we faced off in the trapezoid of light trickling from my bedroom. The next thing I knew, the doorman forced his face through that fragment of light and pressed his lips to mine.

I flooded with panic. How could this be happening *again*? The force of the incident shoved that mental cardboard box from its dusty shelf, spraying its contents across the dim hotel corridor. I racked my brain: What had I done to give the impression that this was okay?

I tried to pull away but the doorman placed his hand at the back of my head and pulled me firmly into his embrace. Just like that night on Megabus, I manually shifted into survival mode and allowed my mind to wander on autopilot.

Safety first, I told myself. Better raped than dead, I told myself.

After what felt like days but was probably only a few minutes, the jovial and playful doorman released my face without warning. He looked me over and I shamefully averted my gaze. I couldn't tell you how I looked or what I was thinking or how we parted ways. But we did.

I went out of my way to avoid The Doorman for the rest of my stay but to no avail. He must have been able to tell that I was upset. Maybe he was afraid I'd tell on him because, for whatever reason, he went out of his way to be nice to me every day for the rest of my stay. One time, while opening the front door for me, I think he even tried to apologize.

I don't really remember because, as I have on so many other days, after he finally left me alone, I crawled around the hotel corridor doing what I could to gather up the contents of my mental cardboard box. I replaced what I could find and added as much of that particular evening as would fit. I crammed the lid on top and wrapped a rubber band around the middle for good measure. Then, I pretty much tucked that box back on its shelf until today.

I don't know why I'm telling you all this shit. It feels rude to rummage through my mental cardboard box when I'm sure you've got one of your own. I don't dig through this box very often. But these memories are congested in my chest, and when I try to breathe through them in meditation, I can't help but cough up the phlegm.

My survival has hinged upon slut-shaming myself into silence. I told myself I got what I deserved.

What you do with your mental cardboard box is your business, but I'm tired of hiding my pain at the bottom of a box. I'm allowed to feel my shame *and* my anger *and* my sadness *and* my frustration *and* my guilt *and* my malice *and* my vindictiveness *and* my hatred *and* my bloodlust *and* my grief. There's space for all of it because that's what being human is about. It's about surviving your nightmares and daring to dream again.

I think just trying to do that is more than enough. In fact, I'm sure it's plenty. In the end, my struggles are always a gift because they reveal the strength inside of me.

A year or two ago, on a hot-ass night about midway through July, I decided to ride my scooter to my girlfriend's house on the other side of town. The wind lashed against my skin as I whipped through the muggy night. A few minutes later, my front tire clipped an unmarked hole in the road. I was pitched off my bike and thrown through the night. The scooter's full force merged with the side of my body, my rib cage grating on the pavement. I remember thinking, "So *this* is what it feels like to be a wheel of Parmesan cheese."

I don't remember how my helmet broke, or when my face got drenched in quite so much blood. But what I vividly recall from beneath my shock was a deep sense of irony. I giggled and thought, "Are your arms still too fat, Jessamyn?"

Near-death isn't the only way to debilitate self-hate, but it's not a terrible place to start. Because really, there's nothing that can facilitate self-love quite like pondering whether your interior organs are still intact. I'd almost recommend it were it not for the residual trauma and medical bills.

In my quest to determine whether or not my body is worthwhile, I forgot that only necrophiliacs think corpses are sexy.

Hating myself is a reflex of getting to know myself. In my self-hate, I see the reflections of those who've hurt me and those who hurt them. I see the necessity of my pain and the futility of avoiding it. Everyone is doing the best they can with the cards life deals them, including everyone who hurts me.

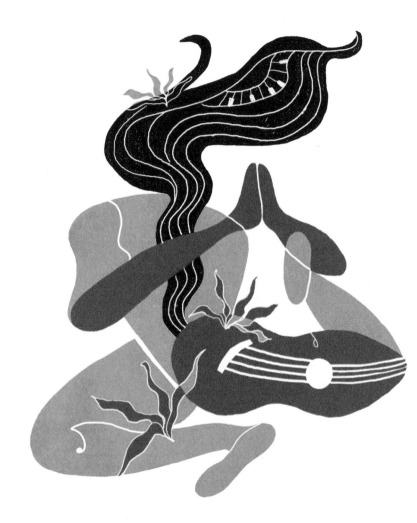

SACRED
MUSIC
& PLANT
MEDICINE

"Changing all these world situations is not in our hands. We are not going to stop all these things. But what is in our hands is the ability to find joy and peace right here and now. If we live in the present, even though the whole world might blow up in a minute, it won't bother us. We can be happy in situations of tension . . . To be happy this minute is in our hands . . . And a smile costs nothing. We should plague everyone with joy. If we are to die in a minute, why not die happily, laughing?" (Satchidananda, 128)

Sometimes, the only way I can deal with my anxiety is by smoking weed and listening to music. Music and weed set me straight. They soothe my soul and make it possible for me to return to myself.

Music has always been my one true love. Singing was how I learned to express myself. Singing is how my ancestors survived. My mother and my aunts were always singing and my Grandma Marvella loved to sing. They say my Great-granddaddy Fred was always singing, too.

Grandma Marvella sang all the time—mostly spirituals, but other stuff, too. She revered music, and all kinds of music at that. But she never sang just *any* song: She always sang *her* song, her own unique melody. She had a very particular tenor range that I haven't heard since she died—it was utterly unique. She sang harmonies that died with her.

She had this really particular way of singing "Amazing Grace." It was unlike anyone else's and it felt impossible to harmonize with. It was infuriating, actually. I wanted her to sing the way I knew. I wanted her to fit into what I could understand. But she didn't give a fuck about what I wanted because she was singing her song. She was playing her instrument. And she taught me to play my own.

Now, my Grandma Emmalou has the greenest thumb you've ever seen. She can grow anything anywhere, anytime, anyplace. She still lives up the road from where my family was enslaved and she has devoted her life to her land. She grows her garden of tobacco, tomatoes, and yams. One time she even ran over her own foot while mowing her lawn and then DROVE HERSELF TO THE HOSPITAL.

My grandmas taught me all I know about sacred music and plant medicine. That both are necessary for you to grow. My Grandma Marvella never kept much alive beyond African violets and I don't think I've ever heard Grandma Emmalou sing in my life, but that's why you have two grandmas, isn't it?

Music is prana in action. It flows across time, space, and intersections, carrying memories, dreams, fears, love, and sorrow. And regardless of genre, secularity or religion, all music is sacred music. Tchaikovsky, Tupac, and Insane Clown Posse all express the spiritual life force that flows from and through each of us.

Music sets my yoga practice on fire and my playlists are sentimental rollercoasters stitched together by memories. Music is powerful medicine, and it guides you to a deeper connection with your breath, but it can also distract you from your breath, which is really the most important music of all. And sometimes it's hard for me to make music with my own instrument when I'm distracted by whatever random playlist my teacher has decided to play during class.

That's why I rarely listen to music when I practice yoga postures with other people, especially if I'm practicing with brand-new practitioners. When you're learning to play your *own* instrument, external music can be extremely distracting.

But once you make a solid connection with the instrument inside of you, listening to sacred music holds you down. It can be in your head or on Spotify, but pick music that provokes your memory, and the more random the better. Sew your playlists together like a patchwork quilt. Use scraps of memories from the different parts of your life and your different identities. Each scrap will flow through your body, reintroducing you to yourself.

I know some people curate yoga playlists based on genre or specific artists, and Lord knows I love a good Beyoncé playlist as much as the next person. But my yoga music has to run like water, and I can't be hemmed in by genre. I think sacred music should run through you like a river of memories, each one pushing you deeper inside yourself.

My favorite yoga album is Kendrick Lamar's *good kid, m.A.A.d city*. K-Dot wrote about the yoga of his life, the yoga of his youth in Compton, the yoga of his decision-making, the yoga of his grief and sorrow. He and I don't have the same story, but in his authentic truth I hear my own. And when I hear his music during my practice, I find my way back to myself.

Yoga and weed have a relationship that's thousands of years old, and more than anything, it guides you to a deeper connection with your breath. But I don't remember the first time I smoked weed. It was so long ago and, truth be told, I've smoked so much since then that it's really asking a lot for me to call up that particular memory. All I really remember is that it happened in a well-manicured park in the rich kid part of Winston-Salem when I was in high school. I was with a pack of friends from my theater class, including a girl from my physics class that I'd been crushing on since day one of junior year. Our squad shared a J of reggie and, if I'm thinking of the right night, I pretended to be a little paranoid so my companions would think I was *really* high. I had no idea what it meant to be *really* high beyond the symptoms my friends told me about in advance, so when it came time for me to take my hit, I just concentrated on not coughing up either of my lungs and pretending to be paranoid if anybody asked.

I was curious about smoking weed, but I really wasn't all that interested. I definitely wanted to seem cool in front of my friends, but that was about it. If memory serves, at least one of them was in a band, which was the pinnacle of all mortal coolness for a hipster coming of age in the early aughts. Between my tatted Chuck Taylors and the fact that I was definitely breaking my boarding school curfew, I was feeling pretty cool and I wanted to make sure everyone else thought I was, too.

But I really wasn't sold on our chosen activity. I mean, I was definitely committed to the whole "being a rebel" thing, and smoking weed in a park seemed like the textbook definition of cool on the surface. And by that I mean it seemed like something Betty Rizzo would've done in *Grease*.

But according to what I vaguely recalled from my fifth-grade D.A.R.E. classes, "marijuana" was the devil's lettuce, and it might make me either froth at the mouth or try to stab someone. Or was that PCP? I couldn't quite recall all the details, but I knew it'd probably be a bad scene. It didn't seem like any of my very cool and rebellious park friends had ever stabbed anyone, but who knew? Maybe I'd be the first in our crew to be a walking statistic.

I was convinced that weed was dangerous until well into college, and I didn't start smoking regularly until my very early twenties. And even then it was only because my girlfriend would bring it over to smoke before sex.

Yoga really changed my relationship to weed. I was still unsure about whether or not it was the devil's lettuce, but in the early days of my yoga practice I started smoking weed right before going to class. When the yoga started kicking my ass, the weed made it infinitely easier for me to be patient with myself. More than feeling high, I felt healed.

Before I started smoking weed regularly, I was a little bit angry and anxious all the time. It got to the point where I thought I was *supposed* to feel that way. I thought smoking weed would tranquilize my senses and distort my connection to reality. But capitalism tranquilizes your senses in a way that weed can't. Capitalism makes you cling to the belief that you're fundamentally unworthy and that the right product is out there, somewhere, to bring about evolution. It makes you hungry for something other than what's happening inside yourself. But cannabis unlocks a world beyond capitalistic greed in which you're able to enjoy right now, today. A world in which you're allowed to be yourself.

Smoking weed helps me manage my anxiety so I don't waste my life worrying about shit that doesn't matter. Some people use prescription drugs, but I like to use weed. Smoking weed makes it easier to accept myself and it makes my yoga practice more expansive and transformative. It helps me find a sense of humor toward my cultural appropriation, racism, fatphobia, and slut-shaming.

I know a lot of people don't like to use weed because it makes them feel out of control. Good. You need to lose control. Control is overrated. Control is ruining your life. Control is supremacy in action. Get loose. Be yourself. Divest from the machine and do your thing. Smile for no fucking reason whatsoever. Smile from deep inside yourself. Find a joy that no one can take from you. That's what the weed's for. Finding your smile by any means necessary.

When I smoke weed before practicing my postures, breathwork, or meditation, I'm *so* much more open to what the practice of yoga offers. Yoga is tough spiritual medicine and cannabis helps it go down A LOT smoother. I'm less likely to throw a temper tantrum when shit gets hard, both on and off the mat, if I regulate my endocannabinoid system.

Honestly, I'm not saying that weed is for you. But I know it's for me. And if you've found another way to deal with the decay of humanity then please, for the love of all that is holy: Get into that shit while the gettin's still good. But would you mind cranking up the music and passing back the blunt on your way out?

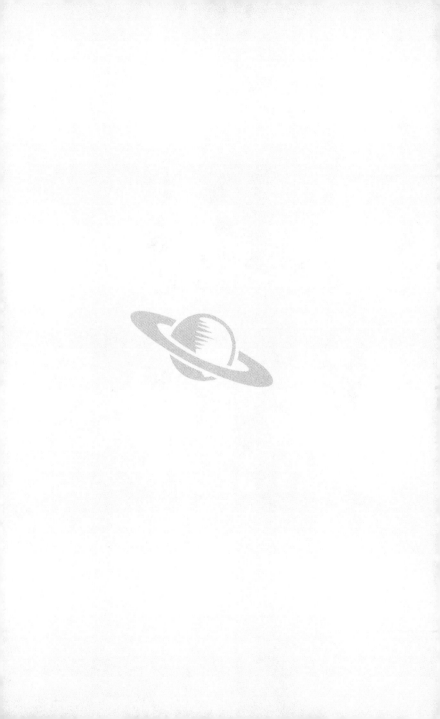

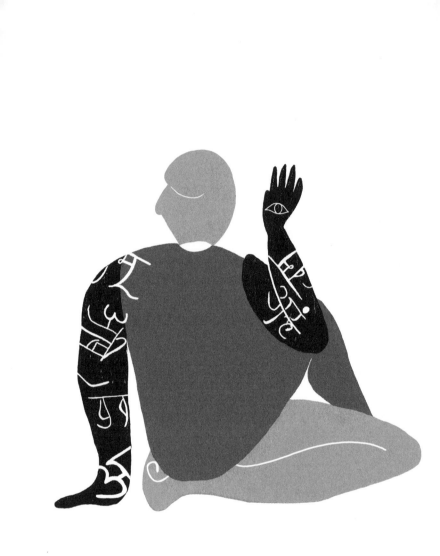

MAMA ALWAYS SAID NEVER TRUST A WHITE BOY

3.52 - "The Yogi should neither accept nor smile with pride at the admiration of even the celestial beings, as there is the possibility of getting caught again in the undesirable." (Satchidananda, 190)

The summer after *Every Body Yoga* came out, I drove up to Asheville to take a workshop led by one of my favorite teachers. This guy has profoundly impacted how I teach yoga. He's really the most body-positive yoga teacher I've ever had, and he's a thin, six-foot-tall, bald White guy. More than anyone else, he's taught me that teaching yoga isn't reciting facts about postural alignment.

He's shown me that teaching yoga is about reflecting your own yoga practice to other people. It's not about recitation or convincing other people to mimic you. It's about authentically embodying your spiritual journey. I've had other teachers, great teachers, but none of them have inspired me like he has.

When I saw that this teacher was leading a workshop about the roots of yoga on one of the rare weekends when I wouldn't be hustling my book, I blacked out the dates in my calendar as quickly as possible.

I'm not the only person who reveres him, and when I entered the yoga studio on the first day of the workshop, there were only a few spots remaining where you could easily roll out your yoga mat. I looked around the room and peeped a spot at the end of the front row, right next to the window. I made my way over and rolled out my mat and supplies, grateful to have snatched up such a low-key spot. I knew my presence wouldn't be easy to ignore. My social media following was pretty big by then and I was one of very few (if not the only) fat Black bodies in the room. I was eager for a spot where my Cancer shell could blend into the scenery as much as possible.

I was really embarrassed by my professional success as a yoga teacher, particularly considering the relatively short period of time I'd been practicing and teaching. Sometimes I feel like I'm too big for my britches, and I was critical of how my internet persona has influenced other people to believe that they should worship yoga poses. I felt ashamed of myself and I just knew my favorite teacher must feel the same way.

The workshop was about the philosophical fundamentals of Classical yoga and the first couple of days were pretty uneventful. We translated chunks of Sanskrit passages from *Hatha Yoga Pradipika*, and as a former student of classical Greek and Latin, I was pretty excited to geek out in another ancient language while also nerding out about yoga.

However, by the end of the second day, I had misgivings about the way my favorite teacher talked about yoga. He talked about Classical yoga as though it's a source of ancestral cultural lineage for American yoga practitioners. But as much as I respect and appreciate Classical yoga's lineage, I don't consider it to be my own. Classical yoga, the Vedas, and Sanskrit are rooted in South Asian culture, with particular connective tissue in Hinduism, Buddhism, and Jainism, among many other faiths. I know that many Black American yoga practitioners feel an ancestral connection to Kemetic yoga's North African roots, but I don't. We all come from the cradle of civilization, but *my* ancestral lineage feels very Black, very Southern, and exceedingly American. It felt deeply appropriative and problematic to approach Classical yoga and Sanskrit from the angle my teacher suggested because it made me feel as though I was being told to steal someone else's cultural identity and nullify my own.

I kept trying to explain away my misgivings by reminding myself of two things. One: My teacher *never* said that our individual ethnic and cultural identities were unworthy of self-exploration. Two: Maybe he believes spiritual nonduality renders the duality of our individual cultural identities irrelevant.

Nonduality basically means that even though you and I live in our own meat suits, our meat suits are really just small parts of one collective meat suit, and the collective meat suit is nothing without us and in turn our individual meat suits are nothing without it. Nonduality means that our differences are really just a matter of subjective perception, and that cultural appropriation and racism are insignificant by comparison to our collective existence. White yoga people love using this argument to gaslight people because it wallpapers over sticky conversations about American yoga's history of cultural appropriation and racism.

I've got no quarrel with the theory of nonduality, but I find it to be wholly ignorant of American yoga's reality. American yoga is tied up in American history, which is infected by colonial racism, sexism, genocide, xenophobia, and imperialism. Emphasizing the theory of nonduality lets the legacy of American history cast a shadow over American yoga's future. I felt my teacher was advocating for the necessity of whitewashing American yoga culture.

I was so distracted by this train of thought that by the end of the third day, I found it impossible to focus on my teacher's lecture. Every time he said something that rubbed me the wrong way, I'd look around the room to see if I was the only person having a visible negative reaction. Everyone else seemed to be nodding in agreement, as though they, too, felt an ancestral connection to Classical yoga. I remembered what happened the last time I brought up cultural appropriation in a yoga class and I thought about not saying anything, but my Virgo rising just couldn't keep her mouth shut. The next time my teacher called for questions, my hand shot in the air.

When my teacher called on me, I swallowed a few times before asking if I was correct in thinking that he believes we're culturally connected to Classical yoga's lineage? And if I *did* have it right, what did he suggest if someone didn't see themselves as a Classical yoga practitioner?

My teacher's face turned to stone and my Virgo rising started to panic. Already this was turning out just like the last time. I filled the echoing silence by babbling about how my question came from my respect for

Classical yoga's integrity and how I felt uncomfortable identifying it as my cultural ancestral lineage.

When I finally stopped jabbering, the room's silence pressed against my eardrums. My teacher narrowed his eyes and the edges of a smirk scuttled across his mouth. He spoke slowly and deliberately, looking me straight in the eye. My fragile bravado shrunk beneath the fearlessness of his gaze. He wanted to make sure I heard his words.

He took a deep breath and told me in no uncertain terms that I probably didn't feel a connection to Classical yoga's lineage because I didn't know enough about the practice in general. I opened and closed my mouth like a trout. He blinked once, and then turned his head to take the next question.

Embarrassed is a bit of an understatement. I felt like he'd backhanded me into next week. I was awash with imposter syndrome. The same imposter syndrome I felt when I got the email about the yolk typo in *Every Body Yoga*. It felt like he'd spoken on behalf of everyone in the world who agreed that I am *way* too big for my britches.

I looked out the window and put my body on autopilot. I let my teacher's words and the emotions they wrought wash over me. I considered the sheer breadth of all the yogic knowledge I didn't yet and might not ever know. I thought about the ways in which I agree with him. That I don't know enough. That I will never and could never know enough. I let the taste of all that roll around in my mouth, under my tongue, and in between my teeth.

Then, I thought about everything I *did* know. And that was when I decided to walk out of the workshop.

I didn't want to cause a scene by walking out in the middle of his lecture. But as soon as my teacher announced our next break, I packed up my shit. I waited for the rest of my classmates to leave the room before approaching him. He and I stared at each other and I averted my gaze to The Floor. I gave The Floor a mumbled excuse as to why I needed to leave before the final day. My teacher listened patiently, waiting for me to stop talking to The Floor. Then he smiled and said he was sorry I needed to leave but that it had been very good to see me and he looked forward to seeing me in the future. I smiled back, walked out of the room, and haven't seen him since.

I should have known that we would have different opinions about cultural appropriation of Classical yoga's heritage. The man's arms are covered with Sanskrit tattoos, for Christ's sake. Plus, in my opinion, White American yoga practitioners like to nullify their cultural identity. I think it's because they're ashamed of the racist legacy of their ancestors. Maybe it's easier for them to pretend it doesn't exist than to deal with the generational emotional fallout.

Looking back, I desperately needed this experience. I hadn't realized it, but I'd pinned all of my spiritual hopes and dreams on the identity of my favorite teacher. I'd cast him in the role of yogic deity and convinced myself that he and I needed to share the same opinions. I don't even think I'd ever really considered him to be human, with his own opinions. But that's the trouble with following other people. It's not his responsibility to be my personal patron saint of yoga. It's not his responsibility to believe in my version of the Truth. We can agree to disagree. Just as he'd done in the past, my teacher taught me how to practice yoga by authentically living his own. Teachers hold up mirrors, and my teacher held up a mirror and forced me to see the truth.

Teachers don't need to cosign your beliefs. They push you to inquire *why* you believe. My anger and frustration facilitated a powerful learning experience, a much more powerful experience than anything I could've expected, an experience that (clearly) continues to this day. He is still my teacher, even though I haven't seen him in years. Our absence from one another is part of how he is teaching me. All the lessons can't happen on a yoga mat. They won't all bloom from love of your teacher. Some of the most important lessons will only happen *because* you hate your teacher.

You'll never know who'll teach you. The best teachers don't even think they're teachers. The best teachers are the ones who piss you off and put you in your place while pushing you out of your comfort zone. They don't think you're hot shit and they're probably unimpressed by what you do. The most important teachers are the ones who lead you to the teacher inside of you.

🦋

Now that I'm finally at the end of this thing, I've started questioning everything. Is this book really good enough? Do I really mean everything I said? Did I leave any of my truth on the floor? And if I did, am I willing to let that truth stand, move forward, and get on with it?

Maybe I should've waited longer to write this book. Waited for more perspective, more knowledge, more distance from this version of my truth. But that's my imposter syndrome, at it again. Just like that night in my office. Still creeping in around the edges. My imposter syndrome, refusing to let me be great.

This imposter syndrome and me, we're just gonna have to kiss and make up. Yes, I will know more later. Later, I will feel different. But later isn't right now, and right now is just as important as later. Right now is the goal, the destination, the only answer.

That's my yoga, my very own church of what's happening now. A quivering, shimmering, trembling collision of contradictions.

What I know for sure is that I'm a beginner and that's all that matters. I don't have to know everything or know more than anyone else. All I can ever do is know myself and that will be enough.

I think not knowing everything can stop you from ever starting anything, but it doesn't have to. You can do what you want right now, today. You don't have to wait for anyone else's approval. You'll never know everything. But that doesn't mean you're not meant to shine bright.

There'll never be enough facts for me to memorize and regurgitate. There will always be someone ready to disagree with or compete with my knowledge. I have to find the courage to be wrong, own it, and move on.

I'm enough. Exactly as I am right now. I don't need to know more or do more or be different at all. I'm a beginner, not an imposter. A beginner doesn't know any more or any better, and a beginner treats everyone like a teacher because a beginner is taught by every body.

I never need to be intimidated by anyone because everyone has something to teach me.

THANK YOU

To ashe and Samantha, for holding me down.

To Mommy, Daddy & Gabriel, for pointing me north.

To Maisie, for standing in the muck with me.

To Shanée & Joelle, for reflecting your light.

To Jane, for making it happen.

To Sami & Anna, for having my back.

To Mary, Jocelyn, Chaz, Melody, Mona, Amber, Tori & Molly, for rowing this boat with me.

To Becky, Kim, Barbara, Rebecca, Chloe, Ilana & Moira, for blessing my words with your gifts.

To Kim, Michael, Stephanie, Shala, Libby, Kathryn, Elena, Diane, Anna, Amy, Mooji, Sara, Philip, Elizabeth & Stefanie, for teaching me.

To Sharon Gannon & David Life, for living your yoga and showing me how to live mine.

To Sri Swami Satchidananda, for carrying the torch and lighting the way.